ADHD
PARENTING
MADE SIMPLE

The Complete Guide on how to Manage Behavioral Problems
and Prevent Outbursts in ADHD Children: Understand your
Child's Needs and Prepare Them for a Bright Future

GREGORY STIDE

Also Written By Gregory Stide

THE ESSENCE OF POSITIVE THINKING

An Easy Guide to Using Personal
Empowerment and Optimism as Keys to
Success, Happiness and Stress-Free Living

Contents

ADHD Parenting

Made Simple

The Complete Guide on How to
Manage Behavioral Problems and
Prevent Outbursts in ADHD
Children: Understand Your child's
Needs and Prepare Them
for a Bright Future

GREGORY STIDE

INTRODUCTION

*I*n the journey of parenting, especially parenting a child with ADHD, information is power. *ADHD Parenting Made Simple* is more than just a book; it is a compass to guide you through the often turbulent but rewarding journey of raising a child with ADHD. Our purpose is to empower you, the parent, with a deep understanding of ADHD and to arm you with innovative strategies to create a supportive, nurturing environment for your child.

This comprehensive guide delves into the complexities of ADHD, offering clear, accessible information and practical advice. We aim to simplify the vast amount of research and theories into actionable insights that make a real difference in your daily life. With empathy and expertise, we navigate the challenges and celebrate the unique strengths of children with ADHD. This guide's core is a crucial theme: harmonizing understanding with guidance. It is not just about managing ADHD but about fostering an environment where your child can cope and flourish.

Recognizing that each child with ADHD is unique, we know that a universal solution will not suffice. Instead, this book is designed to equip you with the knowledge and adaptable strategies to meet your child's needs, ensuring they receive the compassion and structure necessary for their personal growth and success.

We focus on a holistic approach, considering not only the child's needs but also the family dynamics and the broader social context.

We provide a balanced perspective that acknowledges the challenges while highlighting the opportunities for growth and learning that ADHD can bring. As we dive deeper into the layers of ADHD and the varying needs of children affected by it, you will gain insights and strategies that will transform your approach to parenting. We start with the basics – understanding what ADHD is and is not. Then, we will explore its science, debunk common myths, and understand its impact on family dynamics. We address the emotional and behavioral aspects, discussing how ADHD affects self-esteem, social skills, and learning.

From there, we will journey into recognizing and embracing your child's uniqueness, tailoring approaches to their personality, and fostering an environment that supports their growth and development. We'll also look at the crucial role of schools and educators in providing guidance on advocating for your child's needs in educational settings.

Prepare to embark on an enlightening journey, one that promises not just to educate but to inspire. Let us uncover together the layers of ADHD and learn to see the world through your child's eyes. This book is not only a resource but a source of hope and encouragement. It's written with the belief that with the proper support and understanding, every child with ADHD can thrive. We invite you to join us in this exploration, to gain new perspectives, and to discover the joys and triumphs of parenting a child with ADHD. Welcome to ***ADHD Parenting Made Simple.***

CHAPTER ONE

UNDERSTANDING ADHD

*I*n the dynamic and often challenging world of parenting, navigating the complexities of Attention-Deficit/Hyperactivity Disorder (ADHD) presents a unique set of challenges and opportunities. Recent data from the CDC indicates that approximately 9.8% of children between the ages of 3 and 17 in the United States have been diagnosed with ADHD, a condition that not only impacts the lives of these children but also profoundly affects their families, educators, and communities. Understanding ADHD is crucial for turning these challenges into opportunities for growth and positive change. In the late 18th century, Sir Alexander Crichton described symptoms resembling ADHD, noting children with a *"remarkable incapacity of attending."* This early recognition highlights the longstanding nature of ADHD.

In his book, *ADHD: A History of the Disorder*, Russell Barkley, a leading expert in ADHD, provides a comprehensive historical perspective on the disorder, including its terminology changes and the development of its diagnostic criteria over time. Barkley's work is widely recognized and respected in ADHD research. Barkley outlines the journey of ADHD, which saw significant milestones in the 20th century.

Initially termed *"Post-Encephalitic Behavior Disorder"* and later *"Hyperkinetic Impulse Disorder,"* the condition's understanding evolved from a focus on hyperactivity to include inattention and impulsivity. Including ADHD in the Diagnostic and Statistical Manual of Mental Disorders (DSM) in 1980 marked a pivotal moment. Since then, subsequent editions have refined the diagnostic criteria, reflecting growing knowledge and changing perceptions of ADHD.

SECTION 1: WHAT IS ADHD?

Understanding ADHD in its entire spectrum is a game-changer for parents. It's not just about the occasional inattention or bursts of energy; ADHD manifests in various ways, impacting different aspects of a child's life. This section aims to broaden your perspective, revealing the multiple facets of ADHD symptoms. Such comprehensive knowledge shapes effective support strategies, enabling you to meet your child's specific needs with greater insight and adaptability.

ADHD manifests in a spectrum, from quiet daydreaming, often mistaken for laziness, to impulsive actions that overshadow creativity. These are just a glimpse into the diverse examples that highlight the multifaceted nature of ADHD. The understanding of ADHD has evolved significantly. Initially viewed merely as a behavioral issue, it's now recognized as a complex neurodevelopmental disorder. This evolution, marked by pivotal research and changing perceptions, reflects a growing understanding of ADHD's intricacies.

DEFINITION AND SYMPTOMS

Attention-Deficit/Hyperactivity Disorder (ADHD) is a neurodevelopmental disorder characterized by patterns of inattention, hyperactivity, and impulsivity that impact daily functioning and development. Symptoms can include difficulty focusing on tasks, disorganization, difficulty following instructions, and an inability to remain still. These symptoms vary in their intensity and manifestation, making it essential for parents and caregivers to understand their child's specific experiences with ADHD.

ADHD presents differently at various developmental stages. It might manifest as extreme restlessness and difficulty following simple instructions in preschoolers. School-aged children often display challenges in focusing on classroom activities or completing homework. Adolescents with ADHD might struggle with organizational skills and impulsive behaviors, impacting their academic and social lives.

COMMON MISCONCEPTIONS ABOUT ADHD

ADHD is often misunderstood. It is not the result of poor parenting or indicative of a child being lazy or defiant. Such misconceptions can obscure the real challenges faced by children with ADHD. Misconceptions about ADHD not only spread misinformation but also create challenges that extend beyond the child, affecting the entire family dynamic.

One prevalent myth is that ADHD is simply a lack of discipline or a consequence of inadequate parenting. This misconception can lead to unnecessary guilt and stress among parents, who might feel responsible for their child's symptoms. It also cultivates an environment where the child might be unfairly labeled as 'problematic' or 'difficult,' impacting their self-esteem and social relationships. By confronting these myths with research and expert insights, we can foster a more empathetic and practical approach to supporting individuals with ADHD and their families.

Let us explore common ADHD misconceptions:

1) ADHD is not a real disorder: This myth undermines the legitimacy of ADHD, often leading to judgment and criticism of affected individuals. ADHD has been recognized for centuries, with extensive research validating its existence. Studies indicate clear neurological differences in individuals with ADHD (Matthews et al., 2014), emphasizing its validity as a disorder.

2) ADHD is a disorder that only affects children: Believing ADHD is limited to childhood can prevent adults from seeking help. Research shows that ADHD persists into adulthood in a substantial number of cases (Owens et al., 2015), emphasizing the need for lifelong management strategies.

3) ADHD is over-diagnosed: The notion of over-diagnosis can lead to skepticism about valid cases. Increased diagnosis rates are attributed to better awareness and improved screening methods, not over-diagnosis (Visser et al., 2015).

4) Children with ADHD are over-medicated: This misconception might deter the use of beneficial medications. Studies suggest that ADHD is often under-treated (Connor, 2015), and appropriate medication can be a crucial component of effective management.

5) Poor Parenting Causes ADHD: This belief places undue blame on parents, adding to their stress and guilt. Research indicates that genetic and neurological factors are the primary causes of ADHD (Barkley, 2015; Ellis et al., 2009), shifting focus from blame to understanding.

6) Girls have lower rates and less severe ADHD than boys: Underestimating ADHD in girls can delay diagnosis and treatment. Recent studies reveal that girls with ADHD experience significant impairments, similar to boys, and their prevalence nearly equals that of boys in adulthood (Owens et al., 2015; Hinshaw et al., 2012).

IMPACT OF ADHD ON CHILDREN'S LIVES

The impact of ADHD on children's lives is profound and multifaceted, affecting their academic performance, social interactions, self-esteem, and well-being. Children with ADHD may struggle with forming friendships and may often feel misunderstood. Recognizing these impacts is crucial in providing the proper support and environment for children with ADHD.

Children with ADHD face social and academic challenges in school. Consider the story of Max, a 10-year-old with ADHD. He often finds it difficult to stay seated or concentrate on tasks in class. During group activities, his impulsive comments sometimes lead to misunderstandings with peers. 7-year-old Jake loves interacting with others but often interrupts or can't wait for his turn in games. His eagerness, a manifestation of his ADHD, sometimes results in him feeling left out or misunderstood, illustrating the social impact of ADHD on children.

At home, ADHD can affect daily life skills and family dynamics. Emily, age 8, struggles with following routines at home. Her parents noticed her needing constant reminders to organize her room or complete homework. The influence of ADHD can introduce unique challenges in daily routines, communication, and the emotional well-being of the entire family. For instance, children like Emily, who struggle with organizing and following routines, can inadvertently create stress in the household. Her parents' need to provide constant reminders and supervision can lead to tension and frustration on both sides.

In families with children like Max and Jake, there's often an increased need for patience and understanding. Max's difficulties in class and Jake's challenges with social interaction affect their self-esteem and have ripple effects on family life. Parents may navigate complex emotional landscapes, balancing the need to advocate for their child in school while managing their child's frustration and isolation at home.

If ADHD symptoms are not adequately understood and managed, they can lead to ongoing challenges. For instance, children like Max might face academic difficulties and lower self-esteem due to their experiences at school. Emily's organizational challenges could impact her ability to manage responsibilities as she grows older. Jake's social interactions might remain affected, possibly leading to fewer friendships and feelings of isolation.

Recognizing and understanding these impacts is essential. It enables families to seek appropriate support, develop effective coping mechanisms, and foster a nurturing environment accommodating the child's needs. This mindset is vital in minimizing stress and enhancing the quality of life for the entire family, paving the way for positive long-term outcomes for children with ADHD.

SECTION 2: THE SCIENCE OF ADHD

The science behind ADHD offers invaluable insights for parents. This section explains the neurological underpinnings of ADHD, uncovering how brain function and development contribute to the condition. Understanding these scientific aspects is crucial, as it fosters empathy and equips you with the knowledge to develop effective management techniques. This information forms the backbone of evidence-based strategies, guiding you in supporting your child's unique journey with ADHD. Recent studies reveal new insights into ADHD management, such as the effectiveness of combination therapies. Research also points to the interplay of genetics and environment in ADHD development, suggesting a multi-factorial cause.

BRAIN DIFFERENCES AND ADHD

ADHD is rooted in brain development, with studies revealing variations in brain structure and function, particularly in areas responsible for executive functions. Children with ADHD often exhibit differences in the frontal lobe, which plays a crucial role in attention, organization, and impulse control.

Understanding how brain differences in children with ADHD affect their learning and behavior is critical to supporting them effectively. Imagine the brain as an orchestra, with each section playing a crucial role in creating harmony. In ADHD, some sections of this orchestra, especially those in charge of attention, organization, and impulse control, do not always follow the conductor's lead.

This can look like your child struggling to focus in a noisy classroom or forgetting instructions soon after they are given. It is not that they aren't trying; their brain is just tuned differently. These differences mean they might learn better with more hands-on activities or clear, step-by-step instructions. Recognizing and adapting to these unique brain patterns can make a difference in helping your child thrive academically and socially.

EXECUTIVE FUNCTION AND SELF-REGULATION

Children with ADHD often face challenges in executive functioning, which includes aspects like self-regulation, working memory, and flexible thinking. These challenges manifest in various ways, such as difficulties regulating emotions, planning and organizing tasks, or maintaining attention over extended periods.

Understanding executive function deficits in children with ADHD can be crucial in navigating their daily challenges. For instance, a child might need help with organizing their schoolwork, forgetting to turn in assignments, or becoming easily frustrated with complex tasks. This is not just forgetfulness or lack of effort; it manifests executive function challenges typical in ADHD.

HOW ADHD MANIFESTS DIFFERENTLY IN EACH CHILD

ADHD does not manifest identically in every child. Its symptoms and effects can vary greatly, influenced by age, environment, and temperament. This calls for a tailored approach to each child, recognizing that strategies effective for one child may not be as effective for another.

Emma, a 10-year-old with inattentive ADHD, often found herself lost in daydreams. Her biggest challenge was following through on multi-step instructions, especially in school. During a science project, her tendency to get distracted resulted in her forgetting crucial steps, leading to her experiment failing. This incident was a wake-up call for her parents and teachers. Together, they implemented a color-coded system and visual schedules to help her stay on track. These tools and regular check-ins significantly improved Emma's ability to manage tasks, boosting her confidence and school performance.

Alex, an energetic 8-year-old, struggled with impulsivity. His actions, often without thought, led to frequent conflicts with his classmates. A notable incident was during a group activity where Alex's impulsive reaction caused a disruption, upsetting his peers. Realizing the need for intervention, his parents introduced a reward system to encourage thoughtful actions. They also enrolled him in martial arts, which provided an outlet for his energy and taught him self-control. Over time, Alex learned to channel his impulsiveness positively, improving his social interactions and self-esteem.

These cases highlight the need for personalized strategies. Emma benefits from visual organization, while Alex responds well to physical activity and behavior rewards.

Understanding each child's unique ADHD manifestation is crucial in devising practical, personalized approaches. This tailored strategy ensures that each child copes with their symptoms and thrives in their environment.

SECTION 3: MYTHS vs FACTS

In the world of ADHD, myths abound, and separating fact from fiction is critical. This section aims to dispel common misconceptions about ADHD, ensuring that you, as a parent, are equipped with accurate, reliable information. By debunking these myths, we lay the groundwork for effective ADHD management rooted in reality and scientific understanding. Armed with the truth, you can approach your child's ADHD with confidence and clarity.

DUBUNKING MYTHS ABOUT ADHD

Numerous myths about ADHD contribute to misinformation and ineffective approaches. For example, ADHD is not caused by too much screen time, sugar intake, or a lack of discipline. It is also a misconception that medication is the only treatment option. Understanding and debunking these myths is crucial for a holistic approach to managing ADHD.

Let us explore some of the common myths:

• **Myth 1**: "ADHD is loud and boisterous"

• **Fact:** While ADHD can include challenging and disruptive behaviors, it often manifests in more subtle ways. Experts state that "ADHD can also manifest in a plethora of quiet and subtle concerns. Many of the symptoms and challenges are quiet, disruptive only to the individual struggling." This includes symptoms like inattention and being easily distracted, which are less observable but equally impactful.

• **Myth 2:** "Kids will outgrow ADHD"

• **Fact:** Contrary to the belief that ADHD is just a childhood disorder, research shows it is a life span disorder. The ADHD challenges of an 8-year-old will differ from those of a 38-year-old, but challenges do persist. Brain scans indicate that structural differences in the brain often remain, affecting time management, emotions, focus, and productivity throughout life.

• **Myth 3:** "Medication is a quick fix for ADHD."

• **Fact:** Medication can be part of ADHD management but is not a universal solution. Medication alone can't impact all areas of ADHD, and the effect is not universal. Finding the proper medication and dosage can be a long process, and it should be combined with other science-backed approaches for the best results.

• **Myth 4:** "ADHD is always a standalone issue."

• **Fact:** ADHD often coexists with other conditions. Anxiety, depression, oppositional defiant disorder, learning disabilities, and autism are some of the most common additional conditions that occur with ADHD.

- **Myth 5:** "ADHD can't be improved"

- **Fact:** The concept of neuroplasticity shows that the brain can change and adapt. Neuroscientists have found that structural and symptomatic changes can occur in the brain through specific activities and repetition.

THE TRUTH ABOUT DIET, DISCIPLINE, AND MEDICINE

When it comes to managing ADHD, the roles of diet, discipline, and medication are often subjects of keen interest and, sometimes, debate. Each element plays a unique part in addressing the diverse symptoms of ADHD, offering a multifaceted approach to care.

While these concepts play a role, they are part of a comprehensive approach to ADHD management. A holistic approach, including behavioral therapy, educational support, and understanding family dynamics, is essential for effective management.

Recent studies suggest that while diet alone does not cause ADHD, certain foods may exacerbate symptoms. For instance, a diet high in sugar and processed foods might increase hyperactivity in some children. Conversely, foods rich in omega-3 fatty acids, like fish and nuts, have been associated with improved concentration levels.

Discipline in children with ADHD requires a blend of firmness and understanding. Traditional disciplinary methods may only sometimes be effective due to self-regulation and impulse control challenges. Instead, positive reinforcement, consistent routines, and clear, concise communication can be more effective. Examples include using a reward system for desired behaviors or breaking tasks into smaller, manageable steps. The key is to set clear expectations and boundaries while acknowledging the unique challenges your child faces.

Medication is a well-known treatment for ADHD, often used to help manage symptoms such as inattention, hyperactivity, and impulsivity. Stimulant medications are commonly prescribed and can significantly improve focus and control impulsive behaviors. However, they are not a one-size-fits-all solution and may only suit some children. It is essential to work closely with a healthcare professional to determine if medication is appropriate for your child and to monitor its effectiveness and potential side effects.

THE IMPACT OF ADHD ON FAMILY DYNAMICS

ADHD affects not just the individual child but the entire family. Parents and siblings may face challenges in understanding and adapting to the child's behavior. This can influence family relationships and dynamics. It is not uncommon for siblings to feel overshadowed or parents to experience stress due to the extra attention and resources directed toward the child with ADHD. These dynamics can lead to guilt, frustration, and misunderstanding within the family unit. Acknowledging and addressing the impact on family life is crucial for creating a supportive and nurturing environment.

Providing a supportive home environment, strengthened by open and honest communication, is vital. Encourage family discussions where each member, including siblings, can express their feelings and concerns. This fosters understanding and empathy, helping to alleviate feelings of neglect or resentment. Establish routines and clear expectations, which can be comforting for both the child with ADHD and other family members. Consistency helps reduce uncertainty and conflict, creating a more harmonious home life.

Engaging in activities that include all family members can reinforce bonds. Choose activities that accommodate the interests and abilities of the child with ADHD while being enjoyable for other family members. This shared time can strengthen relationships and create positive memories.

Acknowledging and celebrating the achievements of all children in the family is also essential. This recognition can boost self-esteem and foster a sense of belonging and achievement for each family member. By addressing these challenges head-on and implementing strategies to improve communication, understanding, and support, families can navigate the complexities of ADHD more effectively, leading to more robust, more resilient family relationships.

Embarking on this journey with your ADHD child is an act of courage and love. Understanding ADHD is more than a step; it is a leap toward empowerment. Recognizing your child's unique challenges and strengths transforms your parenting approach and family dynamics. This path requires patience, deep empathy, and an unwavering commitment to learning and adapting.

Embracing the journey with your ADHD child is a process that involves continually deepening empathy and cultivating patience. The challenge lies in recognizing that each day can bring new situations requiring patience and understanding. This part of the journey is about adapting to the unexpected and learning to see the world through your child's eyes, celebrating their unique perspective. Remember, in each challenge lies an opportunity to grow stronger and more connected to your child.

This chapter has set the stage, providing key insights and foundational knowledge. Armed with this understanding, you can navigate the ADHD journey with greater confidence and resilience. The tools and strategies outlined here are your compass, guiding you to create a supportive and understanding environment where your child can thrive.

As we move forward, this book will provide you with practical, actionable strategies tailored to your child's unique needs. From behavior management techniques to nurturing positive outcomes, we will explore ways to harness your child's potential. Each chapter is a step towards a future filled with hope and possibilities.

The path ahead is a long-term commitment. It's about preparing for various life stages, from childhood through adolescence, and adapting strategies to suit evolving challenges. This part of the book will discuss how to anticipate and prepare for these changes, ensuring that your parenting evolves alongside your child's growth. Together, let's build a roadmap that leads to success and fulfillment for your child and your family.

CHAPTER TWO

EMBRACING YOUR CHILD'S UNIQUENESS

*M*eet Annie and Sam, two children with ADHD, yet worlds apart in their behaviors and needs. Annie, a daydreamer, often lost in her thoughts, struggles to focus in class. Her homework is frequently incomplete, not due to a lack of effort but an inability to sustain attention. On the other hand, Sam is the perpetual motion machine, always on the move, interrupting others, and finding it impossible to sit still - two children with two very different ADHD journeys.

In essence, Annie and Sam's stories illustrate that ADHD is not a one-size-fits-all condition; it's a complex tapestry that varies significantly from one child to another. Understanding this diversity is crucial as we explore the intricacies of ADHD and how to tailor parenting approaches to each unique child.

SECTION 1: PERSONALITY AND ADHD

Every child with ADHD has a unique blend of traits and tendencies, and understanding this personal mix is crucial. This section will teach you how to recognize and appreciate how your child's unique personality traits intertwine with their ADHD symptoms. This understanding is critical to developing personalized management strategies that work for your child, not against them, transform-

15

ing challenges into opportunities for growth and self-discovery. Children with ADHD display a wide array of personality types. For instance, some children find solace in art, a contrast to ADHD symptoms. In this case, a parent can use this passion to enhance focus. Extroverted children sometimes express energy that amplifies their impulsiveness, and parents can use this to channel energy into group leadership roles.

IDENTIFYING YOUR CHILD'S TEMPERAMENT

Understanding your child's temperament is the first step in tailoring your approach to their ADHD. Temperament refers to the innate aspects of an individual's personality, such as introversion or extraversion, sensitivity, and adaptability. It significantly influences how ADHD symptoms manifest and how they are managed.

Sarah's eight-year-old daughter, Lily, was diagnosed with ADHD. Initially, Sarah struggled with Lily's frequent daydreaming and inattentiveness. However, upon realizing that Lily was introverted, Sarah shifted her approach. She created a quiet, cozy space for Lily to do her homework and engaged her in one-on-one activities that didn't overwhelm her. This new understanding of Lily's introverted nature led to a significant improvement in managing her ADHD symptoms, helping Lily feel more comfortable and focused.

Children with ADHD often exhibit a range of temperaments. For instance, some may be naturally more reserved and introspective, constantly daydreaming and lost in their thoughts, leading to inattentiveness in structured settings. Others might display a more outgoing temperament, characterized by impulsivity and constant motion. To identify your child's temperament, consider tools like personality quizzes or observe their behavior in different settings – how they interact with others, their response to changes, or their approach to tasks.

HOW PERSONALITY INFLUENCES ADHD SYMPTOMS

Annie's introverted nature and daydreaming are a part of her reflective temperament, affecting her attention differently from Sam's extraverted, impulsive actions. These personality traits guide how ADHD symptoms are expressed and managed. A child with an introverted and sensitive personality might struggle with inattention due to internal distractions and sensitivity to external stimuli. In contrast, an extroverted child might exhibit more hyperactive and impulsive behaviors, seeking constant engagement and stimulation. Environmental factors, such as family dynamics and schooling, also play a significant role in shaping a child's personality and how their ADHD symptoms manifest.

Reflective and sensitive children often get lost in their thoughts, leading to inattentiveness. However, their reflective nature can also mean they're intensely creative. Strategies for these children involve creating structured yet flexible environments that encourage creativity while minimizing distractions.

TAILORING APPROACHES TO PERSONALITY TRAITS

For Annie, structured yet gentle guidance works best, keeping her engaged without overwhelming her. Sam's physical activities and clear, concise instructions help channel his energy constructively. Tailoring your approach to your child's unique personality can make a significant difference.

Creative children might be interested in activities that allow them to express their imagination, such as painting, music, or storytelling. Encouraging these activities helps them to channel their energy positively and productively. Analytical children may display an affinity for structured, logic-based activities. Introducing them to puzzles, strategy games, or STEM-related tasks, like basic coding or science experiments, can stimulate their minds and keep them engaged.

For introverted children, create a calm, structured environment for introspection and gentle engagement. For extroverted children, incorporate more physical activities and opportunities for interactive learning. Resources like tailored activity books, ADHD-friendly apps, and structured play can be helpful. Activities like mindfulness exercises or sports can benefit different personality types, aiding in managing ADHD symptoms more effectively. The key is to match the approach with the child's inherent personality traits.

On the other hand, Jake, known for his boundless energy and extroverted personality, found traditional indoor activities less engaging. Recognizing this, his mother introduced him to outdoor sports like soccer and hiking. These activities provided a suitable outlet for extroverted children and their energy, with a long-term positive impact on focus. Engaging in these physically active pursuits helped Jake enhance his ability to concentrate during more sedentary indoor tasks, striking a balance between his need for movement and quieter activities requiring attention.

SECTION 2: STRENGTHS AND CHALLENGES

ADHD isn't just about the hurdles; it's also about the unique abilities and potential each child holds. This section is dedicated to helping you identify and nurture these strengths while navigating the challenges. We'll explore the critical role of self-esteem in ADHD and how bolstering your child's confidence can create a foundation for success.

Recognizing what they naturally excel at is the key to nurturing a child's talent. This could be a creative skill like drawing, a physical ability in sports, or an intellectual strength in math or science. Observing your child's activities and noting where they spend most of their time or show the most enthusiasm can provide insight into their natural inclinations.

Once you've identified your child's strengths, provide them with the tools and resources to cultivate these skills. This might mean investing in specific educational toys, enrolling them in specialized classes, or simply dedicating time at home for practice. Encourage regular practice and exploration in their area of interest. This consistent effort is crucial for skill development and confidence building.

RECOGNIZING AND NURTURING INNATE TALENTS

Every child with ADHD possesses unique strengths. If channeled correctly, Annie's creativity and Sam's energy can be powerful assets. Recognizing and nurturing these talents provides a foundation for success and self-esteem.

Joshua has always struggled in traditional classroom settings, often feeling restless and unengaged. However, his parents noticed his keen interest in drawing. They enrolled him in an after-school art class, where Joshua's talent and passion for art blossomed. The focus required for his art projects helped him learn to manage his ADHD symptoms better. This newfound outlet not only improved his behavior at school but also significantly boosted his self-esteem. Joshua's story highlights the transformative impact of recognizing and nurturing a child's innate talents.

Children with ADHD often possess unique talents that, when nurtured, can lead to significant achievements. Identifying these strengths involves observing your child in different settings and noting what activities they are naturally drawn to and excel in. For example, a child who shows creativity in storytelling might be encouraged through writing workshops or drama classes. Another child with a knack for dismantling and reassembling objects could be guided toward engineering or mechanics-based activities. Focusing on these strengths boosts a child's skill set, self-esteem, and overall development. By affirming their abilities, parents can help them see beyond their ADHD diagnosis to their potential.

PREPARING FOR DIFFERENT STAGES OF LIFE

Navigating life stages from childhood through adolescence requires adaptability. As mentioned earlier in Chapter 1, transitions may be more challenging for children like Emily and Alex, necessitating proactive preparations and support to ensure they thrive at each stage.

Transitioning through life stages poses unique challenges for children with ADHD. For instance, moving from elementary to middle school might overwhelm a child due to increased academic demands and social dynamics. Parents can prepare their children by discussing what to expect, setting up organizational systems, and advocating for support within the school. During adolescence, emotional regulation and peer relationships become focal points. Here, open communication and guidance in navigating social situations are essential. Expert opinions suggest balancing providing support and encouraging independence to build resilience.

THE ROLE OF SEL-ESTEEM IN ADHD

Building self-esteem is crucial. Celebrate successes and provide reassurance in moments of struggle. A strong sense of self can be a child's best defense against the challenges of ADHD. Recognizing and celebrating every achievement, big or small, is vital in fostering a child's self-esteem and motivation. Whether completing a complex puzzle, performing in a school play, or simply improving in their chosen activity, acknowledging their progress encourages them to keep striving and growing in their talents.

Building self-esteem in children with ADHD is a multifaceted approach. Within the family, consistent positive reinforcement, celebrating small victories, and focusing on effort rather than just outcomes is crucial. In school settings, collaboration with teachers to identify and support the child's strengths, alongside accommodations for their challenges, plays a significant role. Self-esteem built through these channels can lead to long-term benefits, including improved mental health, coping strategies, and a positive outlook. Encouraging children to engage in activities where they can experience success is vital in fostering a sense of accomplishment and belonging.

Nine-year-old Eve faced challenges in maintaining self-esteem due to her difficulties in school. Her parents and teachers collaborated to create a supportive environment for her. They focused on her strengths, like her creativity and curiosity, and provided positive reinforcement. Her teacher incorporated interactive learning activities that catered to Eve's learning style, and her parents encouraged her in home-based projects that aligned with her interests. This approach led to a noticeable improvement in Eve's behavior and self-confidence, illustrating the critical role of supportive networks in enhancing self-esteem in children with ADHD.

SECTION 3: ADHD BEYOND THE DIAGNOSIS

ADHD is more than a label; it's a part of your child's journey that influences various aspects of their life. This section explores the broader impact of ADHD, encouraging you to look beyond the diagnosis. You'll learn how ADHD affects learning and behavior, social interactions, family dynamics, and overall well-being. This holistic understanding is essential for supporting your child fully in all areas of life.

PARENTING GUILT AND ACCEPTANCE

It's common for parents to experience guilt, wondering if they could have done something differently. Embracing acceptance is critical. It's important to understand that ADHD is not a result of parenting but a neurological condition that requires understanding and support.

Linda's journey with her son, Michael, reflects a common narrative among parents of children with ADHD. Initially, Linda was consumed by guilt, constantly questioning if her parenting style contributed to Michael's struggles. This guilt often clouded her ability to respond effectively to his needs. Over time, with support from other parents and a deeper understanding of ADHD, Linda transitioned to a place of acceptance. She realized ADHD was not a fault but a part of Michael's unique makeup. This shift in perspective empowered her to adopt more effective strategies, improving Michael's behavior and their family dynamics.

Parenting a child with ADHD often comes with a unique set of emotional challenges, notably guilt and acceptance. Parents might grapple with feelings of guilt, questioning whether their actions or inactions contributed to their child's condition. This guilt can be exacerbated by societal judgments or comparisons with other children. Overcoming this guilt involves understanding that ADHD is a neurobiological condition, not the result of parenting choices. Acceptance plays a pivotal role – recognizing ADHD as a part of your child's life but not the defining aspect. Embracing the diagnosis opens doors to positive parenting strategies, shifting focus from what isn't working to what can lead to growth and success. Support groups, counseling, and educating oneself about ADHD can aid in this journey toward acceptance and effective parenting.

THE EFFECTS OF ADHD ON SOCIAL SKILLS AND RELATIONSHIPS

Children with ADHD may struggle with social interactions. Developing social skills through practice, role-playing, and guidance can help. Encourage and facilitate positive social experiences and friendships.

Eight-year-old Jamie, diagnosed with ADHD, often found herself isolated at school. Her impulsivity and inattentiveness made it challenging to forge lasting friendships. Her parents, noticing her struggle, worked with a therapist to develop strategies tailored to Emma's needs. They organized small, structured playdates, allowing Jamie to interact in a less overwhelming environment.

They also practiced conversation skills and turn-taking at home. Gradually, Jamie began to build friendships, her confidence grew, and her social skills improved, showing that with the proper support, children with ADHD can develop meaningful relationships.

Children with ADHD often face hurdles in social interactions and forming relationships due to impulsivity, inattention, or hyperactivity. They might interrupt conversations, miss social cues, or struggle with emotional regulation, impacting friendships and peer relationships. Structured social skills training can be beneficial for improving these social skills. Role-playing exercises, social stories, and guided play sessions can help children learn and practice appropriate social behavior. Encouraging participation in group activities or sports where children can interact with peers in a structured environment is also beneficial. Success stories from other parents highlight the importance of patience, consistent reinforcement of positive social behaviors, and working closely with teachers and counselors to support the child's social development.

COMORBID CONDITIONS AND THEIR IMPLICATIONS

ADHD often coexists with other conditions like anxiety, depression, learning disabilities, or autism spectrum disorders. These comorbid conditions can complicate the management of ADHD and require a multifaceted treatment approach. For instance, a child with ADHD and anxiety may need both behavioral therapy for ADHD and therapy or medication for anxiety. Parents must work with healthcare providers to understand the implications of these comorbid conditions and create a comprehensive treatment plan. Strategies may include a combination of medication, therapy, and educational accommodations to manage both ADHD and the co-occurring condition effectively. Regular monitoring and adjustments to the treatment plan, based on the child's progress and changing needs, are essential for managing these complex cases successfully.

In addition to his ADHD diagnosis, Jason also struggled with anxiety, a common comorbidity. His parents noticed that his anxiety exacerbated his ADHD symptoms, creating a challenging cycle. Working closely with healthcare professionals, they developed a comprehensive plan that included behavioral therapy for ADHD and anxiety-specific strategies. They also created a calm, predictable home environment and used relaxation techniques to help Jason manage his anxiety. This tailored approach not only helped Jason cope with his ADHD but also significantly reduced his anxiety, leading to improved overall well-being and academic performance.

Grasping the uniqueness of your child's ADHD journey is more than an act of recognition – it's a foundation for building a stronger bond and a more effective way of communication. This deep understanding paves the way for empathetic interactions and equips you with the insights necessary to address your child's needs. As we close this chapter on embracing your child's uniqueness, we prepare to step into the realm of communication strategies.

The next chapter will delve into the art of effective communication tailored for children with ADHD. Here, we will explore how your newfound understanding of your child's unique world can transform how you talk, listen, and connect with them, enhancing their growth and your relationship. This journey of understanding is a gateway to a more harmonious and fulfilling family life.

CHAPTER THREE

COMMUNICATION BREAKTHROUGHS

*P*arenting a child with ADHD brings unique challenges and opportunities, especially when it comes to communication. Active listening is a cornerstone in this journey, not just as a skill but as a pathway to enter your child's world. This section delves deeper into the nuances of active listening, underscoring its role in fostering a profound connection between parent and child. We aim to unfold layers of this vital skill, illustrating how it transcends mere conversation and becomes a bridge to understanding, empathy, and stronger emotional bonds. Through practical strategies and real-life examples, we'll see how active listening reshapes interactions, turning everyday conversations into opportunities for growth and mutual understanding. This section is not just about honing a skill; it's about transforming how you connect with your child, ensuring they feel heard, valued, and deeply understood.

SECTION 1: LISTENING SKILLS

Effective communication with your ADHD child starts with listening. This section will teach you active listening skills to better understand and connect with your child, turning potential conflicts into bonding and mutual understanding moments. In the realm of parenting a child with ADHD, mastering active listening is akin to unlocking a new level of understanding and empathy.

ACTIVE LISTENING AND ADHD

Active listening is more than hearing words; it's about understanding the message your child is conveying. It involves paying full attention, acknowledging their feelings, and responding thoughtfully. Successfully mastering active listening involves maintaining eye contact and paraphrasing your child's words to ensure clarity and understanding.

Active listening is a transformative tool in parent-child communication. Consider the case of Michelle and her son, Dylan. During a heated discussion about homework, Michelle listened actively, focusing intently on Dylan's words, acknowledging his frustration, and reflecting his feelings back to him. This approach shifted the conversation's tone, allowing Dylan to express himself more openly and leading to a mutual understanding of his struggles with a particular subject. This example highlights how active listening can change the dynamics of a conversation, leading to more effective problem-solving.

THE ROLE OF VALIDATION AND EMPATHY

Empathy is the bridge that connects your world to your child's experiences. It's about seeing the world through their eyes. This section will guide you on expressing empathy effectively and validating your child's feelings and perspectives, which is crucial for children with ADHD who often feel misunderstood.

Empathy in communication goes beyond mere understanding; it's about genuinely connecting with the child's emotions. Take the example of Mark, who was often reprimanded for being disorganized. Upon realizing how overwhelmed he felt, his mother expressed empathy by sharing her disorganized experiences. This empathetic approach made Mark feel understood and opened a pathway for discussing practical solutions together. Such empathetic exchanges validate the child's feelings and foster a supportive environment for tackling challenges.

AVOIDING COMMON COMMUNICATION PITFALLS

Miscommunications can escalate quickly, especially with children who have ADHD. We'll identify common pitfalls, like interrupting, ignoring, or responding with frustration, and provide strategies to avoid them.

Common communication pitfalls include interrupting, dismissing concerns, or responding with frustration. For instance, when a child talks about their day, interrupting to correct the story's details can make them feel unheard, impacting their willingness to share in the future. Similarly, dismissing concerns, such as saying "It's not a big deal" to a child's worries, can lead to feelings of invalidation. Awareness of and consciously avoiding these pitfalls can lead to more positive and open communication channels with your child.

Let's take the story of Helen and her 12-year-old son, Tyler. One evening, Tyler was struggling with his science project. Feeling overwhelmed, he started to shut down. Helen initially responded with frustration, saying, *"Why can't you just focus and finish this?"* This approach made Tyler more upset and less cooperative. Recognizing her mistake, Helen took a deep breath and changed her approach. She calmly asked Tyler what part of the project was troubling him. By shifting from a confrontational stance to a more understanding one, Helen avoided the pitfall of escalating the situation. This change in her approach allowed Tyler to open up about his confusion, and together, they could break down the project into manageable parts. This example illustrates the importance of avoiding reactive responses that can lead to communication breakdowns.

SECTION 2: VERBAL INTERACTION TECHNIQUES

Effective verbal communication is pivotal in guiding and supporting a child with ADHD. Verbal strategies can minimize misunderstandings and foster a positive and cooperative environment for your child. In the realm of parenting a child with ADHD, effective verbal communication emerges as a cornerstone. This section delves into the nuances of pivotal verbal interaction techniques in guiding and supporting your child. The focus is on how using essential techniques like clear, concise instructions and understanding the impact of tone can minimize misunderstandings and foster a positive and cooperative environment.

EFFECTIVE WAYS TO GIVE INSTRUCTIONS

The art of giving instructions is more than just conveying a message; it's about ensuring it's received and followed effectively. This section outlines strategies to deliver instructions in a way that resonates with a child with ADHD. It emphasizes the importance of repetition, simplicity, and calmness. For younger children, breaking tasks into small, manageable steps is effective, while teens may benefit from a more collaborative approach, such as having input in their homework schedule. Visual aids for household chores are suggested for younger children, while clear expectations and timelines are recommended for older kids. The overarching principle is ensuring that instructions, regardless of the child's task or age, are delivered clearly and concisely.

Tailoring your approach to your child's age and the situation is critical. For younger children doing homework, instructions should be simple and broken down into small, manageable steps. For teens, a collaborative approach where they have input into their homework schedule can be more effective. Regarding household chores, visual aids like checklists can help younger children, while setting clear expectations and timelines works better for older kids. Always ensure instructions are clear and concise, regardless of the task or age.

THE ROLE OF TONE AND VOLUME

Your tone and volume can convey as much as your words while significantly impacting how your child responds. A harsh tone might be perceived as criticism, leading to defensive or upset reactions, while a calm, gentle tone can be soothing and more effective. Knowing how your vocal expressions can influence your child's behavior and emotions is important. For instance, a softer tone can de-escalate a situation, whereas a louder, more assertive tone might be necessary to capture their attention in a noisy environment.

To illustrate, consider a scenario where a child is reluctant to do homework. A harsh, loud tone might cause the child to become defensive or shut down. However, adopting a calm, understanding tone and lowering the volume to invite closeness can make the child feel supported and more willing to engage. Another example is managing behavior in public spaces. A louder, more assertive tone might be necessary to get the child's attention in a noisy playground. Yet, it's crucial that this assertiveness doesn't translate to harshness but rather remains clear and firm, guiding the child effectively without causing distress.

Communication is about more than what is said but how it is said. By mastering the nuances of tone and volume, parents can enhance their ability to communicate effectively with their children, fostering a deeper understanding and a stronger bond.

BUILDING NEGOTIATION SKILLS WITH YOUR CHILD

Knowing how to negotiate is a critical skill in achieving mutual understanding and agreement. There are several strategies to build negotiation skills with your child, helping them feel heard and part of the decision-making process.

Effective negotiation involves a balance between listening and expressing your views. Start by presenting the issue non-confrontationally, then listen to your child's perspective. For example, if the issue is reducing screen time, explain your concerns about balance and health. Ask for their input on how they think it can be managed. Together, find a middle ground that respects both your concerns and their interests. This step-by-step approach encourages cooperation and teaches valuable life skills in problem-solving and communication.

Laura, the mother of 12-year-old Max, faced challenges with her son's excessive screen time. Concerned about its impact on his sleep and homework, Laura addressed the issue through calm and clear communication. One evening, she initiated a conversation with Max, maintaining a gentle tone. She explained her concerns and the need to set boundaries for his screen time.

Instead of dictating rules, Laura involved Max in the discussion, asking for his input on what he thought was a fair amount of screen time on school nights. They agreed on a reasonable limit and a system for earning extra screen time during weekends for good behavior. This collaborative approach helped set clear boundaries and made Max feel respected and involved in decision-making, enhancing his compliance and understanding.

SECTION 3: NON-VERBAL CUES

Beyond words, the subtleties of non-verbal communication play a crucial role in connecting with your ADHD child. Here, we discuss the significance of body language and facial expressions and how they can bridge or create communication gaps. This section offers insights into using non-verbal cues to reinforce your messages and create a nurturing atmosphere for your child.

UNDERSTANDING AND USING BODY LANGUAGE

Often, what's not said is as important as the words spoken. Body language, such as posture and eye contact, affects communication, and you can use it to enhance your interactions with your ADHD child. For example, a misunderstanding arose due to a mother's unintentional stern body language. While discussing a recent school performance with her daughter, the mother's furrowed brows and crossed arms made her feel criticized, leading to her shutting down and not participating in the conversation. Realizing this, the mother consciously tried to soften her expressions, uncross her arms, and maintain a more open posture in future discussions. This change in non-verbal communication helped her daughter feel more at ease, leading to more open and effective conversations.

Research indicates that body language significantly influences communication, especially with children who have ADHD. Non-verbal cues like posture, eye contact, and proximity can either comfort or distress a child with ADHD. For example, leaning forward slightly can show interest, while crossed arms might be perceived as disapproval. Experts suggest using open, relaxed body language to foster a more receptive communication environment with ADHD children.

THE IMPORTANCE OF FACIAL EXPRESSIONS AND GESTURES

Facial expressions and gestures are integral to non-verbal communication, especially in interactions with children with ADHD. They can either forge a more profound connection or inadvertently create barriers. This expanded section delves into the nuances of facial expressions and gestures conveying understanding, empathy, love, and support.

Children with ADHD often rely heavily on these non-verbal cues to interpret the tone and intent of conversations. A parent's warm smile, an encouraging nod, or a gentle touch can provide reassurance and foster a sense of security. Conversely, a frown, a dismissive wave, or an impatient tap can be misinterpreted, leading to misunderstandings and emotional disconnect.

However, it's just as important for parents to be attuned to their child's non-verbal cues. A child's slumped shoulders might indicate disappointment, while averted eyes could signify discomfort or avoidance. Recognizing these subtle signals can help parents understand their child's emotional state and respond appropriately. Understanding and consciously utilizing facial expressions and gestures can significantly enhance communication and emotional connection with a child with ADHD. This mindfulness, coupled with the ability to read and respond to the child's non-verbal cues, is a powerful tool in nurturing a strong, empathetic, and communicative relationship.

IMPACT OF ENVIRONMENTAL FACTORS IN COMMUNICATION

The environment plays a crucial role in communication. A calm, organized space can aid in more transparent communication. Creating a conducive environment for effective communication with your ADHD child can be accomplished in several ways. First, the setting in which communication occurs can significantly affect its effectiveness.

Furthermore, creating a conducive environment for communication involves more than just a physical space. For serious discussions, a quiet, private space can help a child with ADHD focus on the conversation without distractions. Open spaces that allow for movement can be beneficial for casual interactions. The key is to adapt the environment to suit the nature of the communication and the child's needs.

The Smith family faced challenges in communicating effectively with their son, who has ADHD. They decided to designate a quiet corner in their living room for discussions to improve this. This space, free from distractions and with comfortable seating, became a safe haven for conversations.

The change in environment had a significant impact, making their son feel more relaxed and focused during discussions. This simple alteration in their home setting facilitated better understanding and more meaningful interactions between the parents and their son.

Effective communication is the cornerstone of a solid parent-child relationship, especially when navigating the complexities of ADHD. By embracing these techniques and strategies, you improve communication and foster a deeper bond and understanding with your child.

As we conclude this chapter on crafting an ADHD-friendly home environment, we lay the foundation for our next critical step: building behavior management strategies based on robust and empathetic communication.

With this groundwork in place, we discuss the importance of creating an environment that nurtures and supports the unique needs of a child with ADHD. The upcoming chapter will offer insights and strategies to enhance the home environment further, ensuring it's a place where your child can thrive while feeling safe and understood.

CHAPTER FOUR

CRAFTING AN ADHD-FRIENDLY HOME

*I*magine your home as a garden, a special place where your child, like a unique and vibrant flower, can bloom. Each element in this garden - from the soil to the sunlight - plays a crucial role in nurturing growth. Your home environment acts as this nurturing space, thoughtfully structured to support, engage, and calm, allowing your child to thrive.

Just as a well-tended garden requires care, attention, and thoughtful planning, so does your home environment for your child with ADHD. Think of the peace and beauty a well-maintained garden can bring, and envision that same sense of harmony and growth within your home. Several practical strategies exist to create an ADHD-friendly home that provides structure and flexibility, ensuring your child's unique needs are met. Like a gardener who tends to various plants with different requirements, you can learn how to nurture your child's growth in a tailored and supportive setting.

This chapter will explore practical strategies for organizing your home to reduce distractions and create a supportive space. Just as a garden requires both open areas for growth and shaded spots for rest, your home will benefit from structured yet flexible spaces. From organizing systems that cater to the ADHD mind to routines that provide stability and predictability, each aspect is designed to help your child thrive. We will also discuss creating calming zones, essential for moments of rest and recharge, much like the peaceful nooks of a garden. This chapter is your guide to crafting a living space that complements the unique needs of a child with ADHD, fostering growth, learning, and harmony.

SECTION 1: ORGANIZATIONAL SYSTEMS

Creating an organized environment is critical for children with ADHD. There are several strategies for simplifying and decluttering living spaces, making them more ADHD-friendly. We'll explore using visual aids and reminders to aid daily organization, ensuring tasks and responsibilities are easily visible and understandable. Additionally, creative storage solutions, uniquely suited for the ADHD mind, can be designed to reduce clutter and enhance focus. By implementing these techniques, parents can create a structured yet adaptable environment, crucial for minimizing distractions and helping children with ADHD navigate their organizational challenges more effectively.

SIMPLIFYING AND DECLUTTERING STRATEGIES

Creating a simplified and decluttered environment is especially beneficial for children with ADHD, as it minimizes distractions and promotes focus. This process involves categorizing and organizing items in an understandable way for these children. For instance, using clear, labeled bins for toys can help a child quickly find what they need and put it away, reducing clutter and decision-making stress.

Adopting a minimalist approach to belongings, where only frequently used or favorite items are kept, also helps maintain a calm and orderly environment. Regularly reassessing room layouts, removing unnecessary furniture or decor, and ensuring ample space for movement and play can contribute to creating a peaceful atmosphere conducive to focus and calm. These strategies collectively aim to create an environment that supports the unique needs of a child with ADHD, making daily life more manageable and less overwhelming.

Beyond the basic decluttering strategies, parents can employ color-coding systems for different categories of items, making it easier for children with ADHD to locate and organize their belongings. Introducing *'one in, one out'* rules can help maintain minimalism; whenever a new item is brought into the home, an old one is donated or discarded. Also, creating designated 'drop zones' for frequently used items like school bags and shoes can prevent clutter from spreading throughout the house. For paperwork and art projects, digital archiving can be a space-saving solution. Regular 'decluttering days' can become a family activity, involving the child in the process and teaching them organizational skills. These additional strategies can enhance the living environment, making it more ADHD-friendly and manageable.

VISUAL AIDS AND REMINDERS

Picture a typical morning in your household. There's a rush to get everyone ready for school and work. Amidst the chaos, you may repeatedly remind your child to grab their backpack or put on their shoes. These daily struggles are familiar to many parents of children with ADHD. Visual aids can transform your daily routines, making mornings smoother and your child more independent.

Visual aids and reminders are essential in creating an ADHD-friendly home. Color-coded calendars, for instance, can be transformative. Some families choose to implement a color-coded system in their household. Each family member had a designated color, simplifying scheduling and reducing confusion for an ADHD child. Additionally, color-coded daily routine charts, school materials, and weekly calendars can provide visual cues that make tasks and schedules easier to understand and follow.

When organizing school materials, each subject could be assigned a distinct color. For instance, math materials are in blue folders, while science materials are in green folders. This simplifies schoolwork management. Families may use color-coded stickers or markers on a weekly calendar to indicate events and activities.

For example, appointments are in red, school events are in blue, and extracurricular activities are in yellow.

Reminder boards are another effective tool. They serve as a central point for family communication. Families may opt for a large whiteboard in their kitchen to list weekly tasks and important events. This visual reminder helps children who struggle with forgetfulness stay informed and prepared for upcoming activities. Setting up and maintaining reminder boards can greatly benefit your child with ADHD.

Here are some tips to make the most of these visual tools:

* Place the reminder board in a central, easily accessible location, like the kitchen. This ensures that everyone in the family can see it and stay informed.

* Create a daily routine chart outlining tasks like getting ready for school, chores, and homework. Having a visual checklist reduces forgetfulness.

* List important weekly events, school assignments, extracurricular activities, and family outings. This helps your child plan and prepare.

* Maintain the board by updating it daily or weekly. Encourage your child's involvement in keeping it current.

The emotional and psychological benefits of these visual tools are significant. They instill a sense of accomplishment in your child when they can independently check off completed tasks. This boosts their confidence and self-esteem, reinforcing a positive self-image. Moreover, the precise organization and reduced stress from reminders contribute to a more harmonious family environment. These boards help manage daily tasks and empower your child to take control of their responsibilities.

CREATIVE STORAGE SOLUTIONS FOR ADHD MINDS

Creative storage solutions are pivotal for children with ADHD, like Lucas, who benefit from visually appealing and well-organized spaces. His mother revolutionized his art space with brightly labeled bins, each marked with fun, easily recognizable labels. This made organizing his art supplies enjoyable and turned clean-up into a playful activity. The result was a significant reduction in clutter. Moreover, Lucas found joy in this new system, which made locating his art supplies effortless and frustration-free. Such innovative approaches can transform mundane tasks into engaging activities, enhancing focus and organization skills in children with ADHD.

Lucas's story shows how creative storage solutions can significantly benefit children with ADHD. Like Lucas, many children find joy and motivation in visually stimulating and well-organized environments. For instance, Maya struggled with keeping her schoolwork in order. Her parents introduced a color-coded filing system, where each subject had its unique color. This made finding her work more accessible and added fun to her study time.

12-year-old Ethan, who always misplaced his sports equipment, found success with a personalized storage locker at home. His parents labeled each section for different types of gear, and Ethan decorated it with stickers of his favorite sports teams. This system organized his equipment and instilled a sense of responsibility and pride in maintaining his space.

Such innovative approaches, tailored to the child's interests and needs, can transform organization from a chore to a delightful part of their daily routine. They encourage autonomy and develop essential organizational skills, making daily tasks less overwhelming and more enjoyable for children with ADHD.

SECTION 2: CREATIVE ROUTINES

Routines are the backbone of predictability and structure, which is especially important for children with ADHD. Imagine a morning routine where your child knows exactly what to expect, reducing chaos and anxiety. Picture a structured evening routine that helps your child wind down peacefully, setting the stage for a restful night's sleep. In this section, we'll explore the power of routines in creating stability within your home. You'll learn how predictable schedules can comfort your child, providing a sense of security and reducing stress. We'll also discuss the delicate balance between structured routines and allowing room for spontaneity, ensuring that your child experiences both order and the joys of spontaneity. Additionally, we'll examine the practicality of routine charts, a valuable tool for visual learners, and explore how they can be a game-changer in your child's daily life. These concepts are essential elements of crafting an ADHD-friendly home, and as we dive into them, you'll discover the transformative impact they can have on your child's well-being and your family's daily life.

THE IMPORTANCE OF PREDICTABLE SCHEDULES

Implementing predictable schedules in the daily routine of children with ADHD is very important. Such schedules provide a framework of consistency and security, which is crucial for their well-being. Implementing structured routines for daily activities like mealtimes, homework, and bedtime is not just about maintaining order; it's about creating an environment where children with ADHD can thrive.

These routines help mitigate the anxiety often associated with unpredictability and improve the ability to focus and engage. Moreover, a well-established schedule can foster independence and confidence as children learn to anticipate and prepare for the day's activities. By sticking to a predictable routine, parents and caregivers can provide the stability and structure necessary to help children with ADHD navigate their day with greater ease and success.

Leo, a 9-year-old with ADHD, struggled daily with transitions, which often led to morning chaos and evening meltdowns. His parents, recognizing the need for a stable routine, established a clear, consistent schedule. Breakfast at 7 a.m., homework at 4 p.m, and bedtime at 8 p.m. became predictable pillars in Leo's day. This regularity, much like the reliable rising and setting of the sun, provided Leo with a sense of security and control.

Over time, Leo's anxiety lessened, his focus during homework improved, and bedtime became a peaceful ritual. This example underscores the transformative power of predictable schedules in providing a comforting rhythm to a child's day, much like a metronome guides the tempo of a song.

BALANCING STRUCTURE WITH THE NEED FOR SPONTANEITY

Balancing structure with spontaneity in a child's life, especially one with ADHD, is necessary to maintain the delicate equilibrium of a well-tended garden. Like the trellises and paths in a garden, structure provides direction and support, guiding a child through their daily life with predictability and security. However, just as a garden thrives with areas of wild beauty, children with ADHD also need spaces and opportunities for spontaneous exploration and creativity.

This balance allows them to express themselves freely within a safe and familiar framework. It encourages adaptability, fostering resilience and the ability to navigate both structured and unstructured environments. By thoughtfully combining structured routines with moments of unplanned joy and discovery, we create an environment that is both nurturing and liberating, allowing children with ADHD to grow in all aspects of their personality and abilities.

While Leo follows a structured schedule, his afternoons are left deliberately open. This flexibility allows Leo to choose activities based on his interests, whether building a fort, playing a sport, or painting. This blend of predictability and freedom helps Leo feel secure yet unrestrained, fostering his ability to adapt and thrive. It's a dance between the structured steps and the free-form expression, each equally important in the rhythm of a child's day.

ROUTINE CHARTS AND THEIR EFFECTIVENESS

Routine charts, especially when they are visual or interactive, are powerful tools for enhancing a child with ADHD's ability to adhere to daily routines. These charts are a visual reminder and can track various tasks, from household chores to personal care routines. The effectiveness of routine charts lies in their ability to make responsibilities clear, understandable, and engaging. By breaking down tasks into simple, manageable steps, these charts help children with ADHD focus and complete their tasks with greater independence and achievement. The interactive aspect of these charts, such as checking off completed tasks or adding stickers for accomplishments, provides a sense of progress and motivation, making daily routines less daunting and more rewarding.

The options are endless when choosing a routine chart, each suited to different needs and ages. Picture-based charts work well for younger children, helping them visualize tasks through images. More detailed charts with time slots or checklists can foster a sense of responsibility and time management for older children.

Parents can effectively implement these charts by involving their children in the creation process, allowing them to choose symbols or colors, which fosters a sense of ownership and interest. Regularly updating the charts to reflect changing routines or achievements keeps them relevant and engaging. Most importantly, as per the chart, acknowledging and celebrating when tasks are completed can be a great motivator, reinforcing positive behavior and the value of organization.

SECTION 3: CALMING ZONES

It's a busy evening, and your child has had a long day at school. They're overstimulated, overwhelmed by the day's demands. What if your home could offer them a retreat, a special corner just for them, where they could unwind and find solace? In this section, we'll explore the concept of calming zones – those tranquil havens within your home where your child can find peace amidst the chaos.

In the hectic pace of daily life, a calming zone is a refuge for your child with ADHD. It's a place where they can find solace, regroup, and regain their equilibrium. But how do you create such a haven? We'll walk you through the process, offering step-by-step guidance on designing and organizing calming zones within your home.

We'll introduce you to various sensory tools and aids to enhance these spaces, transforming them into serene retreats tailored to your child's needs. And remember, fostering positive relationships between siblings can play a significant role in the success of these calming zones, and we'll delve into strategies for achieving harmony among your children. It's about creating an oasis of calm within your home, and we'll show you how.

DESIGNING SPACES FOR DOWNTIME

Designing spaces for downtime in your home is like creating a tranquil oasis specifically for your child with ADHD. These areas are safe havens where overstimulation is minimized and relaxation is prioritized. Comfortable seating that invites rest, subdued lighting that soothes the senses, and easy access to calming activities like puzzles, coloring books, or gentle music set the tone for these spaces. Add soft textures or a small indoor water feature to enhance the serene atmosphere.

These dedicated zones provide a respite from the day's challenges and a space where your child can practice self-regulation and find peace, which is crucial for their overall well-being.

Carla transformed a corner of their living room into a 'calm zone' with a comfortable bean bag, a small bookshelf filled with her daughter's favorite books, and a soft lamp. This became Samantha's go-to space after school, where she could unwind and gradually transition from the high-energy school environment to the peace of her home. Here, Samantha found her way to self-regulate, often reaching for a book or a puzzle, helping her to center herself.

This simple yet effective space gave Samantha a sense of security. It became a key part of managing her ADHD symptoms, illustrating the profound impact a thoughtfully designed downtime space can have.

SENSORY TOOLS AND THEIR USES

It's a busy morning, and your child is getting ready for school. But today, something is different. They seem more anxious and restless than usual. As a parent, you're unsure how to help them find calm amidst the morning rush. This is where sensory tools come into play, offering a lifeline in such moments. Sensory tools can transform stressful mornings into serene ones, and by understanding their power, you can tailor them to your child's unique needs. Sensory tools turn chaos into tranquility.

Here are some straightforward strategies:

Expanding the use of sensory tools for children with ADHD is about creating a personalized approach to their unique sensory needs. Weighted blankets, for example, can provide a comforting pressure that mimics a hug, fostering a sense of security and calm. Fidget toys are not just distractions; they offer a constructive outlet for excess energy, helping to improve focus. Soothing music or nature sounds can create a tranquil atmosphere, reducing anxiety and aiding in concentration. When thoughtfully integrated into your child's daily routine, these tools can significantly improve their ability to self-regulate emotions and behaviors.

The key is to observe and understand what works best for your child, as each individual may respond differently to various sensory tools. By offering a range of sensory experiences, you can help your child find the most effective ways to manage their sensory needs and anxiety.

Introducing sensory tools into your child's daily routine involves a thoughtful approach. Start slowly with one or two sensory tools to avoid overwhelming your child. Pay attention to your child's reactions and preferences, which may indicate which tools work best. It's also important to note that families have consistently incorporated sensory activities, such as before bedtime or during transitions. Be open to trying different tools and adjusting their use based on your child's changing needs. Remember, the goal is to provide a supportive environment where your child can thrive.

FOSTERING POSITIVE SIBLING RELATIONSHIPS

Fostering positive sibling relationships in a home where a child has ADHD involves creating shared spaces and activities that promote cooperation and mutual understanding. Encouraging siblings to engage in joint projects can nurture teamwork. Activities that require turn-taking and sharing, such as board games or sports, teach patience and empathy. It's also beneficial to have spaces where siblings can engage in individual activities yet still be in each other's company, fostering a sense of togetherness. Family meetings where each child gets to express their feelings and thoughts can help understand each other's perspectives, strengthening the bond.

Celebrating each child's achievements collectively fosters a sense of unity and mutual respect. These strategies aim not only to accommodate the needs of the child with ADHD but also to enrich the lives of their siblings, creating a harmonious family environment.

Let's consider the story of siblings Matthew and Kiara as an example of fostering positive sibling relationships. Kiara initially struggled to understand her brother's impulsive behavior and constant desire to be busy with his hands. Their parents introduced 'sibling bonding time,' a dedicated period to engage in activities they collectively enjoyed. The family held a meeting and discovered that both Kiara and Matthew were interested in gardening. A section of their backyard was dedicated to planting seeds, and both siblings were involved in the maintenance and upkeep of the garden.

This joint activity helped Kiara understand Matthew's world better and allowed him to learn from his sister's patience and attentiveness. This shared experience taught them teamwork, mutual respect, and the joy of achieving a common goal, strengthening their bond and enriching the family dynamics.

Creating an optimal home environment is just the beginning of your journey in supporting a child with ADHD. The next chapter builds on this foundation, guiding you in navigating the complexities of social skills and public interactions. It's vital in preparing your child to confidently and gracefully interact with the world outside your home.

We'll explore strategies for enhancing communication, understanding social cues, and managing public settings — skills crucial for your child's success and well-being. This journey will empower you with the knowledge and tools to support your child in all aspects of life, ensuring they succeed and thrive in their interactions with others.

CHAPTER FIVE

NAVIGATING SOCIAL WATERS

8-year-old Jack steps onto the bustling playground, a world often overwhelming with its unspoken rules and rapid pace. For Jack, making friends had always felt like trying to solve a puzzle with missing pieces. But on this sunny day, something remarkable happened. As he nervously approached a group of children playing soccer, instead of the usual hesitation, he found a welcoming smile. That day, Jack not only kicked the ball but also kicked down the barriers of isolation, scoring his first goal of friendship.

Jack's breakthrough on the playground is more than just a moment of joy; it's a beacon of hope and a testament to the potential within every child with ADHD. As we delve deeper into this chapter, we will explore the essential skills and strategies that can help children like Jack navigate the intricate world of social interactions. From understanding the subtle art of conversation to managing the complexities of group dynamics, this chapter offers practical, empathetic guidance to empower parents in supporting their children's social journey, turning challenges into opportunities for growth and connection.

SECTION 1: BASIC INTERACTION SKILLS

Understanding and mastering social skills are pivotal in the development of a child with ADHD. By teaching children core principles like empathy and turn-taking, you can set the stage for future meaningful interactions. Jack's journey on the playground mirrors the experiences of many ADHD children as they navigate the complexities of social cues and relationships. The upcoming section examines the foundational skills essential for children like Jack. We'll explore how nurturing empathy and the art of turn-taking can open doors to more fulfilling interactions. Children can safely explore and understand various social scenarios through role-playing, gaining confidence and competence. Additionally, we'll highlight the significance of age-appropriate play, a natural and engaging way for children to learn and practice social behaviors. This section will equip parents with practical strategies to guide their ADHD children towards positive social experiences and relationships.

TEACHING EMPATHY AND TURN-TAKING

Empathy and turn-taking are vital skills for children with ADHD, fostering better social interactions. Parents can cultivate empathy in their children, helping them understand and respond to others' feelings effectively. Successful techniques include emotional labeling and reflective listening. Turn-taking is a crucial aspect of social etiquette. Through simple, engaging activities and games, parents can teach their children to patiently wait for their turn, harmoniously enhancing their ability to participate in group settings.

Consider using storybooks or family photographs as tools to explore emotions. Asking questions like "How do you think this character feels?" or discussing the emotions captured in a family photo helps children understand and label feelings. Similarly, reflective listening exercises, where your child repeats or paraphrases what they heard in a conversation, emphasize understanding and responding to emotions.

Incorporate games that naturally teach turn-taking, such as board games or 'Simon Says.' These activities are enjoyable and instill patience and respect for others' turns. Share personal stories or examples from media that highlight empathy, discussing why empathy mattered in those situations. Remember, children often learn by imitation. Displaying empathy and turn-taking in your daily life and pointing out these moments sets a powerful example for your child to emulate. These strategies, woven into everyday interactions, offer a practical and effective way to reinforce these crucial skills.

ROLE PLAYING COMMON SOCIAL SCENARIOS

Role-playing is an invaluable tool for children with ADHD to practice and internalize positive social behaviors. Children can learn and rehearse appropriate responses by simulating situations such as sharing toys, joining in games, or having conversations. There are several tips for creating these scenarios, providing feedback, and encouraging children to reflect on their role-play experiences, all aimed at boosting their social confidence and competence.

Role-playing is most effective when it mirrors real-life situations. For instance, when sharing toys becomes challenging, parents can create a playdate environment to guide their child in negotiating and compromising. Alternatively, simulating a playground setting at home can prepare your child for joining in games, teaching them to ask to participate and how to handle rejection gracefully. Drawing from your child's experiences can make the lessons more relatable and impactful. Adding props and costumes can also enhance the experience, making it more engaging and memorable.

This method teaches practical skills and allows your child to step into someone else's shoes, fostering empathy and understanding. After each role-play, take the time to discuss with your child what they did well and what could be improved. Asking reflective questions like, "How do you think the other person felt?" helps your child to develop critical thinking and emotional intelligence. Through these discussions, children learn to view situations from multiple perspectives, an invaluable skill in social interactions.

Jack's transformation on the playground was not just spontaneous; it was the culmination of careful and thoughtful preparation through role-playing with his parents. By practicing scenarios like joining in games and sharing, Jack learned how to approach his peers and manage his feelings of nervousness. His parents' efforts in creating these role-playing activities, complete with props and reflective discussions, provided Jack with a safe space to rehearse and understand social interactions. This preparation was instrumental in Jack's ability to confidently step onto that playground and engage with his peers, turning a challenging situation into a successful and heartwarming social triumph.

ENCOURAGE AGE-APPROPRIATE PLAY

Structured playdates, for example, offer a sense of predictability and security, making it easier for these children to engage and interact. Imagine a playdate that begins with a craft activity, transitions into snack time, and concludes with free play – this rhythm helps children with ADHD feel more at ease and in control. Outdoor activities, like nature walks or simple sports, blend physical activity with the serenity of nature, helping to improve focus and reduce hyperactivity. Meanwhile, playful learning, such as using building blocks to teach counting, seamlessly merges fun with education, keeping the child's interest piqued while enhancing cognitive skills.

Finally, real-life role-playing, such as pretending to be a shopkeeper or teacher, helps children understand various social roles and responsibilities, providing a safe space to explore and mimic the adult world. These activities, rich in learning and enjoyment, support the intricate social and cognitive development process in children with ADHD.

SECTION 2: DEALING WITH CONFLICT

In the complex world of social dynamics, conflict is not just inevitable but can be particularly challenging for children with ADHD. Their journey is often marked by impulsive reactions and struggles with emotional regulation, transforming simple disagreements into intricate challenges. This critical section delves deeper into conflict resolution strategies specifically designed for children with ADHD. We'll explore methods to help these young minds understand the consequences of their actions and the profound importance of making amends.

By reframing conflicts as opportunities for growth and learning, we empower parents and children to navigate these turbulent waters with greater skill and understanding. This section is not just about resolving conflicts—it's about transforming them into valuable life lessons that enrich a child's social and emotional development.

CONFLICT RESOLUTION STRATEGIES

Effective conflict resolution is crucial for children with ADHD. There are several techniques that parents can use to teach their children how to navigate disagreements constructively. This includes teaching steps for calming down before responding, using 'I' statements to express feelings without blaming, and actively listening to others' perspectives.

In the conflict resolution journey, calming techniques like deep breathing or counting to ten can be invaluable tools for a child with ADHD. These methods act as anchors, grounding them in moments of heightened emotions. Jack's journey on the playground is a testament to the effectiveness of calming techniques in conflict resolution. He used to get frustrated and was always on the verge of outbursts in social situations. His parents, aware of Jack's challenges in social situations, had been working with him on deep breathing exercises and counting strategies to manage overwhelming emotions.

This practice paid off beautifully on the playground. As Jack felt the familiar surge of nervousness, he employed these techniques, finding a sense of calm that allowed him to approach the other children. This newfound ability to regulate his emotions was key in helping him navigate the social complexities of the playground and ultimately led to his triumphant moment of connection and friendship.

Active listening exercises can also be transformative. In a simple exercise, a child listens to a parent share a story and then repeats what they heard. This practice not only hones listening skills but also teaches empathy and perspective-taking. Through these strategies, parents can build a foundation of understanding and empathy within their children, helping them navigate the complexities of social interactions with greater ease and confidence.

Brainstorming solutions together is a crucial part of conflict resolution, especially for children with ADHD. This process involves sitting down with the child and discussing the conflict calmly, encouraging them to think of different ways to solve the problem. It's important to guide them to consider the perspectives and needs of others involved, aiming to find outcomes that are agreeable to all parties. This method teaches children the value of collaboration and compromise. By involving them in finding solutions, they learn the importance of mutual respect and understanding in resolving conflicts, a valuable skill in all areas of life.

UNDERSTANDING THE ROLE OF IMPULSIVITY IN CONFLICTS

Impulsivity, a common characteristic in children with ADHD, often escalates conflicts unintentionally. Impulsive reactions can lead to misunderstandings and disputes, but there are strategies for parents to help their children recognize impulsive behavior and its consequences. This includes teaching pause-and-think techniques, creating a *'think before you act'* plan, and understanding triggers that lead to impulsive responses, aiming to foster self-awareness and self-regulation in social interactions.

Introducing an impulse control journal offers a tangible way for children to recognize and reflect on their impulsive actions. This self-awareness journey can be further supported by a *'pause button,'* a simple yet effective tool that encourages a moment of reflection before reacting. Parents can lead by example, demonstrating calm and considerate responses in stressful situations. Additionally, establishing a system of cues provides a discreet and immediate reminder for the child to pause and reassess their initial impulsive reaction. Enhancing the child's emotional vocabulary is another key strategy, as it empowers them to articulate their feelings more accurately, reducing the likelihood of impulsive outbursts. Through scenario planning, parents can prepare their children for various social situations, equipping them with strategies to manage potential conflicts.

HELPING YOUR CHILD MAKE AMENDS

Making amends is a powerful step toward resolving conflicts and repairing relationships. Parents can teach their children the value of apologies and restitution. This involves acknowledging mistakes, understanding the impact of their actions on others, and taking steps to make things right. Emphasis should also be placed on the importance of forgiveness, both in forgiving others and seeking forgiveness, as a path to healing and moving forward constructively.

In teaching your child to make amends, guiding them through a heartfelt apology process is key. This involves not just saying 'sorry' but understanding and articulating the mistake and expressing genuine regret. Creative restitution, tailored to the child's age, can make amends more meaningful. A broken toy might be mended together, or a sincere note can follow a hurtful word. Role-playing is also useful, allowing children to practice apologies in a safe environment.

Emphasize the importance of forgiveness in your family conversations, sharing stories that illustrate forgiveness in action. And remember, when your child takes steps to make things right, positive reinforcement from you can deeply encourage their growth and empathy. This approach nurtures a deep-seated understanding of responsibility, compassion, and the power of sincere amends.

SECTION 3: ENHANCING PEER RELATIONSHIPS

This section focuses on the art and science of nurturing positive social connections for children with ADHD. This section is not just about making friends; it's a comprehensive exploration of how to sustain and enrich these friendships over time. We will introduce strategies that help children engage more naturally in social networks and extracurricular activities, vital arenas for social development.

By recognizing challenges such as teasing and bullying that children with ADHD may face, we will also empower parents with insightful techniques and supportive approaches to help their children deal with these situations. These tools are designed to boost your child's social confidence and resilience, enabling them to navigate the social world with a stronger, more assured stance. This section is a roadmap to help your child fit in and thrive in their social circles, building lasting, meaningful relationships.

FOSTERING FRIENDSHIPS AND SOCIAL NETWORKS

Fostering friendships and strengthening social networks for children with ADHD is often difficult. Emphasizing the importance of genuine connections, parents can encourage their children to find and bond with peers who share similar interests and values.

Matthew struggled to connect with peers at school. However, he had a deep fascination with robotics. When Matthew's parents enrolled him in a local robotics club, it opened a new world. Surrounded by other kids who shared the same passion for building and programming robots, Matthew found common ground. They worked together on projects, solving problems and sharing ideas. These shared experiences and interests in robotics laid the foundation for genuine friendships. Matthew's story is a testament to how aligning a child's personal interests with social activities can lead to meaningful and fulfilling social connections.

Interest-based playdates can be a powerful tool for parents seeking to foster their child's social connections. For example, suppose a child is passionate about nature. In that case, organizing a playdate with a nature walk or visiting a botanical garden can be enjoyable and conducive to forming friendships. Additionally, parents can act as social facilitators by organizing small group activities tailored to their child's interests and comfort levels.

This approach allows children to interact in a familiar and engaging setting, making social interactions more natural and less intimidating. To foster Jack's interest in sports, his parents arranged playdates with other children who shared his enthusiasm for soccer. They organized small matches in the local park, allowing Jack to interact naturally with his peers in a comfortable and familiar setting. These sports-themed gatherings nurtured Jack's athletic skills and social connections as he bonded with other children over shared goals and team spirit.

To assist children with ADHD in building their social skills, parents can incorporate fun and interactive exercises into their routine. One such activity involves using conversation starters, a simple yet effective game encouraging children to engage in dialogue. Parents can create index cards with various open-ended questions or prompts, which the child can pick and discuss. This game sparks conversation and helps the child practice initiating and maintaining discussions, a critical social skill.

THE IMPORTANCE OF EXTRACURRICULAR ACTIVITIES

Extracurricular activities offer more than skill development; they are crucial for social growth. electing the right activities that align with your child's interests and strengths is important. These activities serve as dynamic laboratories for social interaction, providing your child with real-life scenarios to practice their social skills. Structured activities provide a safe and predictable environment for social interactions. Team sports, arts, and clubs offer many benefits, enhancing social skills, self-esteem, and a sense of achievement.

For instance, participating in a drama club can help a child understand non-verbal cues and develop empathy by getting into character and understanding various perspectives. In team sports, children learn the value of cooperation, communication, and compromise as they work together towards a common goal.

Selecting the right activities that align with your child's interests and strengths is important. It's not about enrolling your child in every activity available; it's about finding the ones that resonate with their passions and abilities. When children engage in activities they genuinely enjoy, they are more likely to persevere and form meaningful connections with like-minded peers. For example, if your child loves drawing, an art class can be a wonderful platform to bond with fellow art enthusiasts who share their creative spirit.

Structured activities provide a safe and predictable environment for social interactions. Many children with ADHD benefit from structured routines and environments. Extracurricular activities often follow a schedule and clear rules, which can help children feel secure and reduce anxiety. This predictability can enhance your child's confidence in social situations, knowing what to expect and how to navigate them successfully.

Team sports, arts, and clubs offer many benefits, enhancing social skills, self-esteem, and a sense of achievement. Team sports, such as soccer or basketball, teach children valuable teamwork, leadership, and cooperation lessons. Arts and creative clubs encourage self-expression and boost self-esteem as children create and showcase their work. As your child accomplishes milestones and receives recognition for their efforts, it enhances their sense of achievement, contributing to a positive self-image.

Consider the story of Gerard, who joined a local sign language club. He was initially hesitant about participating but soon found solace in the beauty of signing and communicating through this visual language. Through this club, Gerard discovered his passion for sign language and formed meaningful friendships with fellow sign language enthusiasts. Gerard's involvement in the club not only boosted his social skills but also improved his self-esteem and sense of accomplishment. Through the sign language club, Gerard not only learned to express himself in a unique way but also became an advocate for inclusivity and communication accessibility. His journey in the club not only enriched his social life but also left a lasting impact on his self-confidence and the lives of those around him.

By selecting the right extracurricular activities aligned with your child's interests, you provide them with opportunities to grow socially, develop self-confidence, and foster lasting friendships that can be sources of support and joy throughout their lives.

HANDLING TEASING AND BULLYING EFFECTIVELY

Teasing and bullying can be particularly challenging for children with ADHD, as their impulsivity and difficulty regulating emotions may make them more vulnerable to these negative experiences. Parents must equip their children with effective strategies to respond to teasing and bullying while preserving their self-esteem and emotional well-being.

One valuable strategy is to teach your child how to assert themselves respectfully. Encourage them to use *"I"* statements to express their feelings and set boundaries. For example, if a peer teases them, they can calmly say, *"I don't like it when you tease me. Please stop."* Role-playing scenarios with your child can help them practice assertiveness in a safe environment.

Emotional resilience is a crucial skill for children with ADHD. It empowers them to bounce back from negative experiences and maintain a positive self-image. Share stories of individuals who faced adversity and overcame it. Highlight how setbacks and challenges can be opportunities for growth and learning.

Teach your child strategies to manage their emotions, such as deep breathing exercises or a *"cool-down"* technique when they feel overwhelmed. Encourage them to talk openly about their feelings, emphasizing that it's okay to seek support when needed. By fostering emotional resilience, you're helping your child develop the inner strength to handle teasing and bullying confidently.

Collaborating with your child's school creates a safer and more understanding environment. Schedule a meeting with teachers and administrators to discuss your child's needs and potential strategies to address teasing and bullying. Schools can implement anti-bullying programs, provide additional support, and educate classmates about ADHD to promote empathy and inclusion. Additionally, work with the school to identify a trusted staff member your child can turn to if they experience teasing or bullying. Establishing this support system can give your child a sense of security.

By providing your child with these tools, teaching assertiveness, building emotional resilience, and collaborating with schools, you empower them to navigate the challenges of teasing and bullying with resilience and confidence. Remember that your support and guidance are vital in helping your child thrive socially.

As we explore the intricacies of meeting your child's social needs, it becomes increasingly evident how crucial it is to address these challenges in a way that suits their unique strengths and struggles. This realization seamlessly guides us into our next chapter, where we delve into "Discipline and Self-Control." Here, we will equip you with effective strategies to navigate the world of discipline, tailored specifically to the needs of children with ADHD, ensuring a holistic and supportive approach to their development.

Hey There!

How About Making a Difference in Someone's Life?

"The greatest joy in life is doing things for others, without expecting anything in return." - Anonymous

Did you know that people who help others tend to be happier and feel more fulfilled? That's what "**ADHD Parenting Made Simple**" is all about! But to spread this message, we need a little help. And that's where you come in!

Would you be Willing to Help Someone You've Never Met also Benefit From This Book?

Imagine someone a bit like you, dealing with their child that has a severe ADHD condition. That person could really use a guide like "**ADHD Parenting Made Simple**."

We would like every parent to have the knowledge and ability to to help their ADHD child. And the secret to doing that is... well, **you**... spreading the word!

Reviews are like a guiding light for someone searching for help and hope. So, here's how you can help others:

Leave a Review: It's easy and quick!

Just scan the QR code below to share your thoughts on what you think of the book thus far:

Your few words could really help others such as:

A small business owner trying to stay positive under pressure.

An entrepreneur keeping their dreams alive.

An employee looking to find joy in their work.

A client trying to turn their life around.

You could really make someone's dream come true!

Join the "**Caring Club**"

If you love helping, you're already a part of our special group. We're excited to share more positive strategies with you!

Thank you for your kindness and support. Every review brings us closer to helping someone transform their life with positivity. Stay positive and keep spreading joy!

- Gregory Stide

P.S. Sharing is caring! So, if you think this book can help someone else, why not share it? It's a great way to spread positivity and help others.

CHAPTER SIX

DISCIPLINE AND SELF-CONTROL

*P*arenting is a journey filled with diverse challenges and joys. Still, when your child has ADHD, these challenges often take on a different dimension, especially in the realm of discipline. Traditional disciplinary methods, which often rely heavily on punishment and strict rules, may not only be ineffective for children with ADHD but can also exacerbate the difficulties they face. This unique situation calls for a rethinking of conventional approaches to discipline.

This chapter will explore how discipline for a child with ADHD can be transformed from a source of contention into a powerful teaching tool. Here, discipline is not synonymous with punishment. Instead, it's about guiding, teaching, and supporting your child as they learn self-control, responsibility, and decision-making skills.

Raising a child with ADHD means recognizing their inherent need for structure and clear expectations, balanced with compassion and understanding of their unique neurology. These children often struggle with impulse control, staying focused, and regulating their emotions, which can lead to disciplinary challenges that might seem insurmountable. However, with the right strategies and mindset, discipline can be reframed as a positive, nurturing process that empowers your child rather than demoralizes them.

This chapter aims to provide you with the tools and insights necessary to develop a discipline strategy that works for your child and your family. We'll delve into techniques emphasizing positive reinforcement over punishment, the importance of natural consequences, and ways to tailor your approach to fit your child's needs. You'll learn about effective behavioral techniques, including the judicious use of timeouts and alternatives, the role of rewards and incentives, and how to create a behavior modification plan that respects your child's individuality.

Moreover, we will focus on the critical aspect of developing self-discipline in your child. Self-discipline is a crucial skill for all children, but it is especially vital for those with ADHD. We'll explore strategies that help children with ADHD self-monitor, use self-regulation tools effectively, and understand the importance of long-term planning and foresight.

By the end of this chapter, you will be equipped with a deeper understanding and practical methods to guide your child toward better self-control and responsible behavior. Remember, discipline in the context of ADHD is a journey of learning and growth for you and your child. It's about building a foundation of love, understanding, and respect to serve your child well beyond childhood.

SECTION 1: RETHINKING DISCIPLINE

In the journey of parenting a child with ADHD, discipline often becomes a complex puzzle. Traditional views of discipline, primarily focused on punishment and rigid rule enforcement, may not only be ineffective but can also be counterproductive for children with ADHD. Discipline for children with ADHD should be about guidance and learning rather than punishment.

The goal is to help these children understand the consequences of their actions and make better choices in the future. This chapter explores how positive reinforcement can be more effective than traditional punishment. We'll delve into the psychology behind why children with ADHD respond better to rewards and recognition and how you can use this knowledge to foster positive behavior and minimize adverse incidents.

REINFORCEMENT VS PUNISHMENT: WHAT WORKS FOR ADHD?

When it comes to disciplining children with ADHD, the traditional approach of punishment often misses the mark. Punishment can lead to feelings of shame and frustration, and for a child with ADHD, who may already struggle with self-esteem, this can be particularly damaging. Instead, shifting the focus to positive reinforcement can open a new world of possibilities, both for the child and the parent.

Children with ADHD often experience difficulty in processing and internalizing negative consequences. Punishments like scolding or taking away privileges might not change the expected behavior. This is akin to speaking a language your child doesn't understand. Instead, think of positive reinforcement as a bridge, translating your expectations into a language they can comprehend and respond to.

Positive reinforcement involves rewarding desired behavior, making it more likely to be repeated. It's like watering a plant; the more you water it, the more it grows. For a child with ADHD, immediate and consistent rewards for positive behavior can be incredibly effective. This could be as simple as praise for completing homework on time, a sticker chart for daily chores, or a special activity after a week of good behavior at school. Each child is unique, so what motivates one child might not work for another. Extra screen time might be the ultimate reward for one child, while another might prefer choosing what's for dinner. It's about finding what sparks joy in your child and using that as a lever for positive behavior.

When a child with ADHD receives positive reinforcement for

good behavior, it creates a feedback loop. They feel accomplished and valued, which boosts their self-esteem and encourages them to repeat the behavior. This positive loop is much like a snowball rolling downhill, gathering momentum and size; each act of positive reinforcement makes the next one even more effective.

Some examples of positive reinforcement in action include:

Behavior Chart: Create a chart where good behaviors are rewarded with stickers. Once a certain number of stickers is reached, they earn a reward. This visual representation of progress can be incredibly motivating.

Immediate Verbal Praise: When your child does something well, immediately praise them. This immediate reinforcement helps them connect the positive behavior with the reward.

Reward Systems: Establish a system where good behavior earns points, which can be exchanged for a bigger reward, like a trip to the park or a small toy. This teaches the value of working towards a goal.

Special Time with Parents: Sometimes, the best reward is time spent with you. A game night, a walk, or a special outing can be powerful motivators.

While focusing on positive reinforcement, it's also important to address negative behavior. Instead of punishment, redirect your child to a more appropriate activity or use logical consequences directly related to the behavior. For example, if a child is not playing nicely with a toy, instead of taking it away as a punishment, guide them to play with it appropriately, reinforcing the right way to use it.

Shifting from punishment to positive reinforcement isn't just about changing your child's behavior; it's about changing your perspective as a parent. It's about guiding, supporting, and celebrating your child, helping them grow into their best selves. Remember, for a child with ADHD, positive reinforcement isn't just a discipline strategy; it's a language of love and understanding.

THE CONCEPT OF NATURAL CONSEQUENCES

One of the most effective ways to teach children about the impact of their actions is through natural consequences. This approach allows them to learn from their experiences in a safe and controlled environment. The concept of natural consequences is a powerful tool in the parenting toolbox, especially for children with ADHD. Unlike artificial consequences imposed by parents (like time-outs or privilege removal), natural consequences are the organic outcomes that follow a child's actions. They are life's way of teaching what happens due to choices made, providing a practical and memorable learning experience.

For example, if your child refuses to wear a coat on a chilly day, the natural consequence is that they will feel cold. This experience teaches them the importance of dressing appropriately for the weather. In contrast to a lecture or punishment, this consequence directly links the child's decision to the outcome, making the lesson more impactful and memorable. To effectively use natural consequences, it's important to ensure that the consequence is safe and that the child understands the potential outcome of their choice.

Here are a few scenarios where natural consequences can be an effective teaching tool:

Homework Responsibilities: If your child chooses not to do their homework, the natural consequence might be receiving a low grade or feedback from the teacher. This teaches the importance of responsibility and the direct impact of their actions on their academic performance.

Cleaning Up Toys: Suppose your child plays with toys but doesn't put them away. A natural consequence would be not being able to find their favorite toy the next time they want to play. This experience teaches them the value of organization and caring for their belongings.

Social Interactions: If a child with ADHD interrupts others frequently, they might find that their peers are less willing to engage in conversation with them. The natural consequence teaches the importance of listening, waiting, and taking turns.

As a parent, your role is to help your child understand the link between their actions and the natural consequences. This might involve some discussion before or after the consequence has occurred. For instance, if your child feels cold after not wearing a coat, you might discuss with them how their choice led to their discomfort and how they might make a different decision next time. It's also crucial to differentiate between natural consequences and neglect. Ensuring your child's safety is paramount; natural consequences should only be used when they are safe and age-appropriate. For example, letting a young child experience the natural consequence of not eating might not be appropriate due to health risks.

A helpful metaphor for natural consequences is the process of gardening. Just as plants need water, sunlight, and care to grow, children need guidance, experience, and understanding to learn. Just as watering a plant leads to its wilting, neglecting certain responsibilities produces natural consequences. This metaphor can help children understand that their actions, like caring for a plant, directly affect the outcomes they experience.

Natural consequences not only teach immediate lessons but also help children with ADHD develop long-term skills like foresight, understanding cause and effect, and self-regulation. This approach fosters independence and responsibility, preparing them for the complexities of adult life where consequences are often natural and self-imposed. Using the concept of natural consequences gives your child a real-world understanding of how their actions affect themselves and others, promoting a deeper sense of awareness and responsibility. This approach, blended with love and guidance, helps children with ADHD navigate their world more effectively, understanding that every action has a reaction, just as in the world around them.

COPING MECHANISMS FOR PARENTS

Parenting a child with ADHD is like navigating a ship through ever-changing seas. One moment, the waters may be calm, and the next, you find yourself amidst a storm. As the captain of this ship, it's crucial to have the tools to maintain your course, ensuring both your well-being and that of your child. Here, we explore coping mechanisms for managing stress and creating a harmonious and supportive environment conducive to your child's growth. Parenting a child with ADHD can be a rollercoaster of emotions and challenges. Parents must have coping mechanisms to manage their own stress and emotions. There are strategies to help you maintain patience, stay calm, and provide consistent and effective discipline. These coping mechanisms are vital for your well-being and creating a stable and supportive environment for your child.

Rethinking discipline in the context of ADHD involves a paradigm shift – moving away from traditional methods focusing on compliance and punishment towards techniques that build skills, understanding, and positive behaviors. By the end of this section, you'll have a deeper insight into how to approach discipline as a constructive and supportive process, laying a foundation for your child's growth and success.

Embrace the 'Pause-and-Reflect' Technique: Before reacting to a challenging situation, take a moment to pause and reflect. Imagine your reaction as a stone thrown into a pond; the ripples affect more than just the point of impact. Ask yourself: *"Will my response escalate or defuse the situation? Am I addressing the behavior or my child's character?"* This moment of introspection can be the difference between a constructive conversation and a heated argument.

Establish a Self-Care Routine: Just like the instructions on an airplane to put on your oxygen mask first before helping others, self-care is vital. Carve out time for activities that rejuvenate you – a quiet coffee break, exercising, or reading a book. Remember, a relaxed and healthy parent is better equipped to handle the demands of parenting.

Develop a Support System: Parenting a child with ADHD can feel isolating at times. Build a network of support comprising friends, family, or support groups for parents of children with ADHD. Sharing experiences and strategies with others who understand can be immensely comforting and informative.

Use the 'Step-Back' Strategy: In a stressful situation, physically step back. This simple action creates a physical and psychological space, allowing you to view the situation more objectively. It's like stepping back to see the forest rather than just the troublesome tree.

Practice Mindfulness and Meditation: Mindfulness and meditation can be powerful tools in managing stress and anxiety. Even a few minutes a day can significantly impact your overall well-being. Picture your mind like a sky – thoughts and feelings are clouds passing by, and you don't have to hold onto them.

Embrace Imperfection: Understand and accept that there will be imperfect days. Like a mosaic, where each imperfect piece contributes to a beautiful picture, each challenging day is part of the journey. Embrace these imperfections as part of the growth process for you and your child.

Set Realistic Expectations: It's easy to fall into the trap of expecting too much from yourself. Remember, parenting is not about perfection. Set realistic goals for yourself and your child. Celebrate the small victories, as they are stepping stones to larger successes.

Seek Professional Help When Needed: There's no shame in seeking help from a therapist or counselor. Sometimes, an outside perspective can provide new strategies and insights, helping you navigate the complex waters of parenting a child with ADHD.

Rethinking discipline in the context of ADHD is not just about changing strategies but our entire approach to parenting. By taking care of yourself, you are setting the stage for a more positive, calm, and effective way of guiding your child. Remember, in the symphony of parenting, your well-being is as crucial as the notes you play to guide your child.

SECTION 2: BEHAVIORAL TECHNIQUES

After rethinking the concept of discipline for children with ADHD, it's crucial to translate this understanding into practical strategies. In this section, we delve into the realm of behavioral techniques that are not only effective but also empathetic to the unique needs of children with ADHD. These techniques are about more than just managing behavior; they teach skills and foster an environment where your child can thrive. As we delve into these behavioral techniques, remember that the ultimate goal is to empower your child, helping them to navigate their world with increased confidence and capability. Let's explore how these strategies can be effectively implemented in your daily life.

EFFECTIVE USE OF TIMEOUTS AND THEIR ALTERNATIVES

Timeouts are a common disciplinary tool in many households, but their effectiveness can vary, especially when dealing with children with ADHD. When used correctly, timeouts can teach children self-regulation and allow them to calm down. However, it's crucial to understand the nuances of implementing timeouts effectively and to be aware of alternative methods that may be more beneficial for children with ADHD.

Clear Communication: Before a timeout is ever used, explain to your child what it is and its purpose. It's not a punishment but a chance for them to pause and collect themselves. Make sure they understand that a timeout is a consequence of specific behaviors, not a reflection of your love or their worth.

Consistency and Predictability: Consistency is critical.

Timeouts should be a predictable response to certain behaviors, not a surprise or something that happens out of frustration. This consistency helps your child understand the cause-and-effect relationship between their actions and the timeout.

Duration: A good rule of thumb is one minute of timeout for each year of the child's age. For a five-year-old, a five-minute timeout is appropriate. Longer timeouts can lead to boredom and frustration, which are counterproductive.

Timeout Spot: Choose a spot that is quiet and free from distractions but in a safe area where you can still monitor your child. This shouldn't be frightening or isolating but a neutral zone for cooling down.

Post-Timeout Discussion: After the timeout, it's essential to have a calm discussion with your child. This is a chance to discuss what happened, why the timeout was necessary, and how similar situations can be handled differently.

While timeouts can be effective, they are not always the best option for children with ADHD, who may struggle with time perception and self-regulation. Here are some alternatives:

* Instead of sending your child away, have a 'time-in.' This involves sitting with your child in a calm area and talking through their emotions. It's about connection rather than isolation, helping them understand and regulate their feelings.

* Sometimes, a physical outlet is more effective than a timeout. If your child is feeling restless or agitated, encourage them to engage in a physical activity like jumping on a trampoline, running around the yard, or even doing a quick set of jumping jacks. This can help them burn off excess energy and regain focus.

* Create a 'relaxation corner' in your home with comforting items (like soft pillows, stress balls, or coloring books). Guide your child to this space when they feel overwhelmed or need a break.

This approach teaches self-regulation by encouraging them to recognize and respond to their needs for calm.

* Teaching your child simple mindfulness or breathing exercises can be a valuable tool for self-regulation. These techniques can help them calm their minds and bodies, especially during stress or overstimulation.

* Sometimes, redirecting your child's attention to a different, more acceptable activity can prevent the escalation of negative behavior. This redirection should be subtle and present a positive alternative to the behavior leading to a potential timeout.

Incorporating these methods requires patience and experimentation to see what works best for your child. The goal is not to enforce discipline but to guide your child in learning self-control and emotional regulation. By using timeouts effectively or employing these alternatives, you can provide your child with the tools they need to manage their behavior constructively and affirmatively.

THE ROLE OF REWARDS AND INCENTIVES

Rewards and incentives can motivate children with ADHD to adopt desired behaviors. We'll delve into how to set up an engaging, fair, and effective reward system. In navigating the waters of parenting a child with ADHD, rewards, and incentives can serve as a beacon of motivation, guiding them toward positive behavior and away from the rocky shores of impulsivity and distraction. This section delves into setting up an engaging, fair, and effective reward system tailored to the unique needs of a child with ADHD.

Children with ADHD often struggle with delayed gratification. A reward system provides immediate and tangible feedback that is more impactful for them. It's like spotlighting the behavior you want to encourage, making it more noticeable and appealing to your child.

Here are some tips to help you design an effective reward system:

* Start by identifying specific behaviors you want to encourage or discourage. For example, completing homework without reminders or playing gently with a sibling. Be as clear and specific as possible – ambiguity can be a hurdle for a child with ADHD.

* Rewards should be given soon after the desired behavior. This immediate reinforcement strengthens the connection between the behavior and the reward in your child's mind. Think of it like watering a plant right after it's been exposed to sunlight – the combination of both leads to growth.

* Use a variety of rewards to maintain interest. These can range from extra screen time, a favorite snack, to a special activity with a parent. Changing rewards periodically keeps the system fresh and engaging.

* Consider a scaling system where small achievements earn smaller rewards, and bigger achievements earn more substantial rewards. It's like climbing a ladder – each step upward leads to a higher reward.

* Involve your child in choosing the rewards. This gives them a sense of control and investment in the system. It's akin to letting them choose the destination on a treasure map.

* Consistently apply the reward system. Inconsistency can confuse your child and reduce the effectiveness of the system.

Imagine your child struggles with completing homework. You could set up a sticker chart where each completed assignment earns a sticker. Collecting five stickers might earn a small reward, like choosing the movie on movie night, while 20 stickers could lead to a bigger reward, like a trip to their favorite park.

While rewards are effective, it's also important to foster intrinsic motivation – the desire to do something for its own sake. Praise and encouragement can be powerful motivators, especially when focused on effort and perseverance. Celebrate the process, not just the result. For instance, praise your child for consistently sitting down to do homework, not just for getting all the answers right.

Incentives promise future rewards and can be particularly effective for longer-term goals. For instance, if your child struggles with morning routines, you might set an incentive like a special weekend activity if they manage to get ready on time each day of the week. Think of yourself as a gardener and your child as a plant. Just as different plants need different amounts of sunlight, water, and nutrients, children with ADHD require different types of motivation and reinforcement. Your role is to find the right combination that helps your child thrive.

Rewards and incentives are not about bribery; they are tools to guide and teach. When used thoughtfully, they can be incredibly effective in helping your child with ADHD develop positive behaviors, like a gardener finding the right conditions for a plant to flourish. Remember, the ultimate goal is to gradually shift from external rewards to intrinsic motivation, nurturing a self-driven and confident child.

CREATING A BEHAVIOR MODIFICATION PLAN

A behavior modification plan can provide structure and clear expectations. Here, you'll learn how to create and implement a plan tailored to your child's needs, helping them achieve better behavior outcomes. A behavior modification plan is like a roadmap for positive behavior change. It provides structure, sets clear expectations, and establishes a consistent framework for you and your child. Creating a behavior modification plan involves understanding your child's unique needs and motivations, setting achievable goals, and using consistent, positive reinforcement to guide behavior. Let's explore how to create and implement an effective plan.

Before diving into the plan, understand your child's specific challenges and what motivates them. Children with ADHD often struggle with impulse control, attention, and following instructions. Observe your child in different settings to identify patterns in their behavior. For instance, does your child have more difficulty following instructions in the morning or during transitions? Understanding these nuances is crucial for tailoring the plan to their needs.

Set specific, measurable, achievable, relevant, and time-bound (SMART) goals. For example, instead of a vague goal like *"behave better,"* opt for something more tangible, such as *"complete homework before playing video games."* These goals should be achievable and broken down into smaller steps if necessary. Think of this as setting up small signposts along the road, guiding your child towards the desired behavior.

As previously discussed, incorporate a reward system to motivate and encourage positive behavior. Choose rewards that are meaningful to your child and appropriate for the behavior you want to encourage. For instance, if your child completes their homework on time for a whole week, they might earn a special activity or a small treat. The key is immediate and consistent reinforcement – like giving a high-five to a marathon runner at each milestone, providing encouragement to keep going.

Consistency is the backbone of any behavior modification plan. It's like watering a plant; regular care leads to growth. Ensure everyone involved in your child's life understands and follows the plan. This consistency helps your child know what to expect and understand the link between their behavior and the outcomes.

Start implementing the plan, focusing on one or two behaviors at a time to avoid overwhelming your child. For instance, start by focusing on morning routines. Use visual aids like charts or checklists to help your child remember what they need to do. Offer praise and rewards immediately after the desired behavior to reinforce it. Regularly review the plan's effectiveness. Like a gardener pruning a plant, adjust the plan to ensure it meets your child's needs.

Celebrate successes, no matter how small, and use setbacks as learning opportunities to refine the plan. As your child masters certain behaviors, gradually increase expectations or shift focus to other areas. This is akin to gradually increasing the weight in a workout routine, building strength over time.

Here are some examples of Behavior Modification Plans in Action:

Morning Routine Plan: If mornings are chaotic, a plan might include a checklist of tasks to be completed before breakfast, such as getting dressed, brushing teeth, and packing a school bag. Each completed task earns a sticker, and a certain number of stickers leads to a reward, such as choosing a weekend activity.

Homework Plan: Set a specific time and place for homework each day. Break assignments into smaller, manageable parts. Each completed part earns a point, and points can be exchanged for a preferred activity or privilege, like extra screen time.

Remember, a behavior modification plan is not a static document but a dynamic tool that evolves with your child's growth and development. It's about guiding them to better behavior, providing support and rewards, and celebrating each step forward. You can help your child develop the skills they need to succeed with patience, understanding, and consistency.

SECTION 3: DEVELOPING SELF-DISCIPLINE

As we journey further into the world of discipline and ADHD, we arrive at a crucial destination: Developing Self-Discipline. While the previous sections focused on external methods of discipline and behavior management, this section focuses inward on the skills and strategies children with ADHD can develop to manage their own behavior and impulses.

Self-discipline is an invaluable skill for any child, but for those with ADHD, it can be life-changing. Children with ADHD often struggle with self-regulation, a challenge that can manifest in difficulty controlling impulses, staying on task, and planning for the future. By teaching self-discipline, you empower your children to take control of their actions, make better decisions, and ultimately lead more successful and fulfilling lives.

In this section, we will explore practical and effective strategies to help your child develop the art of self-monitoring. This skill is pivotal in helping them recognize their own behavior patterns, understand the consequences of their actions, and make conscious decisions to change or maintain those behaviors. These strategies are not just about managing behavior; they are about nurturing a sense of autonomy and confidence in your child, providing them with the skills they need to navigate their world more effectively.

We will also delve into the power of self-regulation tools. These tools, ranging from simple techniques like deep breathing exercises to more structured approaches like organizational aids, can provide your child with the necessary support to manage their emotions and actions in various situations.

STRATEGIES TO HELP CHILDREN SELF-REGULATE

Self-monitoring is a cornerstone skill in the development of self-discipline, particularly for children with ADHD. It involves being aware of one's behavior and its impact and adjusting accordingly. This section offers practical strategies to help your child develop self-monitoring skills, fostering a greater sense of control and responsibility.

Visual aids can be incredibly effective for children with ADHD. Consider using charts or visual diaries where your child can record their behaviors and feelings. For example, a 'behavior thermometer' can visually represent different levels of emotions or actions, from calm to agitated. At the end of the day, review the thermometer with your child and discuss what led to changes in their behavior. This visual reflection makes abstract concepts more concrete and understandable.

Regular check-ins can help your child become more aware of their daily behavior. Set specific times for brief discussions about how they feel they're doing. You might ask, *"How do you think this morning went?"* or *"What could we do differently tomorrow?"* This routine creates a consistent space for self-reflection and planning.

Mindfulness and meditation can be transformative for children with ADHD. These practices teach children to focus on the present moment, recognize their feelings and thoughts, and respond more calmly to situations. Start with short, guided meditation sessions or breathing exercises to help your child learn to pause and assess their feelings and actions.

A token economy system involves earning tokens or points for desired behaviors and losing them for undesirable ones. This tangible system allows children to track their behavior and its consequences visually. For instance, they might earn a token for completing homework without distractions and lose one for interrupting while someone else is speaking. Periodically, they can exchange tokens for a reward, reinforcing the connection between behavior and outcomes. There are also various apps and gadgets designed to aid in self-monitoring. These can range from simple timers that remind your child to assess their current activity or emotion to more complex apps that track behavior patterns over time. Choose tools that align with your child's interests and age.

Journaling or storytelling can be a powerful tool for self-monitoring. Encourage your child to write or tell stories about their day, focusing on moments when they felt proud or faced challenges. This exercise helps them process their actions and the associated emotions, fostering a deeper understanding of their behavior patterns.

Children learn a lot by observing adults. Model self-monitoring by talking about your own experiences. For instance, you might say, *"I noticed I was getting frustrated while cooking dinner, so I took a few deep breaths to calm down."* This shows them how it's done and normalizes the process of self-reflection. Role-playing different situations can help your child anticipate and plan their responses. Create scenarios where they might have to exercise self-control or make a decision and discuss possible outcomes. This practice helps them think through their actions and consequences in a safe, controlled environment.

Help your child set specific, achievable goals related to self-monitoring. For instance, a goal might be to raise their hand and wait to be called on before speaking in class. Celebrate when these goals are met, reinforcing their sense of accomplishment and the effectiveness of self-monitoring. Provide regular, constructive feedback on your child's self-monitoring efforts. Acknowledge their progress, even small, and offer positive reinforcement. This encouragement goes a long way in motivating them to continue practicing and improving their self-monitoring skills.

Incorporating these strategies into your daily routine can significantly enhance your child's self-monitoring ability. Remember, developing self-monitoring skills is gradual, and patience is key. Each small step your child takes in learning to understand and regulate their behavior is a victory in the journey towards self-discipline and independence.

THE POWER OF SELF-REGULATION

Imagine your child's mind as a busy, bustling city. Thoughts are zooming like cars, emotions fluttering like pedestrians, and tasks rising like towering skyscrapers. For a child with ADHD, navigating this city without a map can be overwhelming. This is where self-regulation tools come into play. They serve as the GPS, the street signs, and the traffic lights, helping your child navigate their mental landscape more effectively.

As previously stated, visual aids are powerful tools for children with ADHD. They provide concrete reminders and cues to help these young minds focus and remember tasks. Another effective tool is the use of visual timers. Unlike traditional timers, visual timers display the passing of time in a way that's easy to understand. As the visible portion diminishes, your child gets a clear sense of how much time is left for a task, helping them to manage their activities and breaks better.

Reminder systems act as gentle nudges, helping your child remember and prioritize tasks without feeling overwhelmed. These can range from alarm clocks to set reminders on a phone or tablet. The key is consistency and predictability. For instance, setting a regular alarm for homework time creates a routine that your child can depend on. You can also use physical objects as reminders. A special bracelet or a sticker on their hand can be a physical prompt to remind them to check their planner or to take a deep breath when feeling overwhelmed.

Organizational strategies are like building the framework for your child's daily activities. They provide structure and help reduce the chaos that can be so paralyzing for a child with ADHD. One effective strategy is the use of a Task Board. Create a board that lists daily tasks, divided into 'To Do', 'Doing', and 'Done' sections. This helps your child keep track of what needs to be done and gives them a sense of accomplishment as they move tasks to the 'Done' section. Another tool is the *Chunking Method*, where larger tasks are broken down into smaller, more manageable parts. For instance, if homework seems overwhelming, break it down into individual subjects or sections, allowing your child to focus on one small part at a time.

The key to making these tools effective is integrating them into your daily routine in a way that feels natural. Start by introducing one tool at a time, allowing your child to get comfortable with it before adding another. Involve them in the process—let them choose the calendar colors or their task board's style. This makes it more engaging for them and gives them a sense of control and ownership. Remember, these tools are not just about managing behavior; they're about empowering your child. They provide a way for your child to understand and navigate their world, turning the bustling city in their mind into a well-organized, navigable space.

By incorporating these self-regulation tools, you are not just helping your child manage their ADHD but equipping them with skills that will serve them well throughout their life. In the next chapter, we'll explore how these skills can be further developed and applied in the context of education.

TEACHING LONG-TERM PLANNING AND FORESIGHT

For children with ADHD, the concept of time can be like a river – constantly flowing, hard to grasp, and sometimes overwhelming. Long-term planning and foresight are crucial skills, yet they often elude these young minds that are typically focused on the immediacy of the 'now.' This section provides techniques to help your child envision the future and understand the long-term consequences of their actions, much like planting a seed today to enjoy the shade of a tree years later.

Here are several strategies parents have found helpful:

Use Visual Timelines: Create a visual timeline of activities or goals. This can be a simple calendar or a more creative timeline filled with pictures and milestones. For instance, if your child wants to save money for a new toy, draw a timeline showing how saving a small amount each week adds up over time.

Small Steps for Big Goals: Teach your child to break down large goals into smaller, manageable tasks. If they dream of being in a school play, outline steps like attending auditions, practicing lines daily, and setting aside time for rehearsals. This approach makes a distant goal feel more achievable and less daunting.

Rewarding Milestones: Recognize and celebrate small milestones. This reinforces the value of working towards long-term goals. For a child learning a musical instrument, celebrate learning a new song or practicing consistently for a week.

'If-Then' Thinking: Encourage 'if-then' thinking. Pose scenarios like, "If you do your homework now, you'll have free time this weekend." This helps them link present actions to future outcomes.

Role-Playing Games: Use role-playing games to simulate future scenarios. These games can be fun and educational, allowing your child to make choices and see their 'future' consequences in a safe, controlled environment

Use of Planners and Apps: Introduce tools like planners or digital apps for goal setting and task management. These tools can help your child organize their thoughts and keep track of their progress toward long-term goals.

Reflecting on Past Successes: Regularly remind your child of their past successes. This can be as simple as recalling a time when they worked hard to achieve something. It's a powerful way to show their actions have meaningful impacts over time.

By incorporating these techniques, you are not just teaching your child how to plan for the future but also instilling in them the understanding that their actions today shape their world tomorrow. Like a gardener who plants seeds and patiently tends to them, you are helping your child sow the seeds of their future, nurturing them with the foresight and planning skills they need to flourish.

As we conclude this enlightening journey through the landscape of discipline and self-control for children with ADHD, it's important to reflect on the ground we've covered. We've explored various techniques to help your child learn the art of self-discipline, from understanding and managing their behavior to developing the crucial skill of long-term planning and foresight. These strategies are akin to equipping your child with a compass and a map in a vast forest; they provide direction and guidance, helping them navigate the complexities of life with ADHD.

Remember, instilling discipline and self-control in your child is not a sprint; it's a marathon. It requires patience, persistence, and a lot of love. There will be days when progress seems slow, almost like trying to watch a plant grow in real-time. But with each small step, each moment of understanding and self-awareness your child gains, they are growing stronger, more capable, and more prepared for the challenges ahead.

As we turn the page to the next chapter of this guide, we shift our focus from the foundational elements of discipline and self-control to another vital aspect of your child's development: education. Education plays a pivotal role in the life of a child with ADHD, not just in the academic sense but as a broader concept that encompasses learning, growth, and personal development. In the next chapter, we will delve into the world of education for children with ADHD. We will explore navigating the educational system, advocating for your child's needs, and creating a learning environment that helps them thrive. Education for a child with ADHD is not just about grades and test scores; it's about nurturing their curiosity, embracing their unique way of thinking, and empowering them to reach their full potential.

CHAPTER SEVEN

EDUCATIONAL STRATEGIES FOR SUCCESS

*T*here is a world full of educational strategies that can significantly enhance the success of children with ADHD. Understanding how to navigate the school system and advocate for your child's unique needs is paramount as parents. This chapter equips you with the knowledge and tools to create an ADHD-friendly learning environment that caters to your child's strengths and challenges.

Let's begin with a story that resonates with many families. Imagine a young girl named Sally. Bright, imaginative, and brimming with potential, Sally embodies the spirit of many children diagnosed with ADHD. Yet, like her peers, she found the traditional school environment to be a labyrinth of obstacles. Her innate intelligence and creativity were often overshadowed by her struggles with maintaining attention and managing hyperactivity. These challenges led to a constant battle with the conventional expectations of the classroom setting.

In school, Sally often felt out of place and misunderstood. Her energetic nature and unique way of processing information were considered disruptions rather than aspects of her distinctive learning style. This misunderstanding led to her feeling sidelined, both academically and socially. The lack of support and recognition of her potential left her frustrated and demoralized. However, Sally's story is not one of defeat. It is a narrative of resilience, adaptability, and triumph. Though faced with hurdles, her journey through the education system became a powerful testament to her strength. Sally began to thrive with the support of her parents, who tirelessly advocated for her needs, and educators, who began to recognize and embrace her unique learning style.

The transformation was gradual. It involved creating an individualized learning plan that acknowledged her ADHD, advocating for accommodations that addressed her challenges, and implementing teaching strategies that harnessed her strengths. Sally's parents and teachers worked collaboratively to ensure that her educational experience was not just about managing her ADHD but about enabling her to excel.

Sally's success story is a beacon of hope and a guide. It demonstrates that with the right strategies, understanding, and support, children with ADHD can overcome their educational challenges, excel, and realize their full potential.

As we explore this chapter, keep Sally's story in mind. It exemplifies the core message of this chapter: that with the right approach, every child with ADHD can succeed academically. We will cover various aspects, including collaborating with teachers, effective learning techniques, and overcoming academic hurdles, all geared toward creating a supportive and productive educational journey for your child.

SECTION 1: RETHINKING DISCIPLINE

This section focuses on one of the most critical aspects of ensuring educational success for children with ADHD: building a strong partnership with their teachers. A positive, proactive relationship between parents and educators lays the foundation for a supportive and understanding educational environment. As parents of children with ADHD, one of the most empowering actions you can take is to collaborate with your child's teachers actively. The collaboration between parents and teachers is more than just a series of interactions; it's a partnership that plays a critical role in shaping your child's educational experience and outcomes.When we constantly ponder negative thoughts, it's like adding fuel to an already blazing fire. It stirs stress and apprehension and even contributes to sadness or hopelessness. Conversely, embracing positive thoughts acts like a shield for our mental well-being.

You may be surprised to know that your thoughts and feelings are very closely intertwined. They're like close friends who constantly hang out and do everything together. So, when we cultivate positive thoughts, we also boost our mental health. We feel happier, more resilient, and better equipped to tackle whatever life throws our way.

BUILDING A PARTNERSHIP WITH EDUCATORS

For parents of children with ADHD, creating and maintaining a strong, communicative relationship with educators is not just beneficial; it's essential. This partnership is anchored in mutual understanding, respect, and a shared commitment to the child's educational success. It's about building a bridge between home and school, ensuring that your child's learning journey is supported from both sides.

The first step in building this partnership is establishing open lines of communication. This doesn't mean only touching base at parent-teacher conferences or when issues arise. It involves regular, proactive communication. Share updates about your child's progress at home, ask about their class performance and behavior, and be open to receiving teacher feedback. This two-way communication creates a comprehensive picture of your child's overall experience and needs.

Regular meetings with your child's teachers are vital. These meetings shouldn't be limited to discussing challenges but should also celebrate successes and progress. They provide a forum for discussing strategies, setting goals, and reviewing your child's Individualized Education Plan (IEP) or 504 Plan, if applicable. Consistent meetings help monitor your child's progress and ensure that any necessary adjustments to their educational strategies are made promptly.

A successful partnership is rooted in mutual understanding and respect. Educators bring professional expertise and experience, while you bring in-depth knowledge of your child's personality, habits, and history. Respecting each other's perspectives and expertise is crucial. When educators understand the nuances of your child's ADHD and how it affects their learning, they are better equipped to tailor their teaching methods accordingly.

Involvement in decision-making processes is another critical aspect of this partnership. Whether it's about setting educational goals, choosing intervention strategies, or modifying the learning environment, your input as a parent is invaluable. Being actively involved ensures that the educational approach is tailored to your child's needs.

Finally, consistent support from home and school creates a stable and nurturing environment for your child. This means reinforcing the same values, expectations, and routines in both settings. When children receive consistent messages and support from their parents and teachers, they feel more secure and more likely to thrive. Building a strong partnership with educators creates a supportive network surrounding your child with understanding, encouragement, and the tools they need to succeed. This collaboration is not only about addressing the challenges posed by ADHD but also about harnessing and celebrating your child's unique talents and potential.

INDIVIDUALIZED EDUCATION PLANS (IEPSs) AND 504 PLANS

For children with ADHD, Individualized Education Plans (IEPs) and 504 Plans are critical tools for addressing their unique educational needs. Both are formal plans developed within the school system to provide learning support and accommodations. While they are similar in intent, they differ in scope and the specifics of their services.

An IEP is a more comprehensive plan for students who qualify for special education services under the Individuals with Disabilities Education Act (IDEA). It includes specific educational goals, details about the child's current level of performance, and a tailored plan for services and support. On the other hand, a 504 Plan, named after Section 504 of the Rehabilitation Act of 1973, is designed for students who do not qualify for special education but still require accommodations in the regular classroom. It's often less detailed than an IEP and focuses on providing specific accommodations to help the child learn alongside their peers.

As a parent, your role in developing these plans is vital. Your insights into your child's strengths, challenges, and experiences are invaluable in creating an effective plan. Active participation involves attending and contributing to meetings, sharing observations, and collaborating with educators to develop realistic and achievable goals.

Both IEPs and 504 Plans typically offer the following:

Accommodations: Adjustments in the way lessons are taught or tests are given. For a child with ADHD, this might mean extra time on tests, preferential seating, or breaks during work time.

Modifications: Changes in what a child is expected to learn or know. While more commonly addressed in IEPs, these can also be part of a 504 Plan.

Support Services: These may include access to a special education teacher, speech therapy, or counseling, depending on the child's needs.

Regular Reviews: Both plans require regular reviews and updates to ensure they continue to meet the child's needs.

Understanding these plans and their components allows you to advocate more effectively for your child. It empowers you to ask informed questions, make requests based on your child's specific challenges, and ensure that the school provides the necessary accommodations or modifications. Remember, these plans are not set in stone; they can and should be revised as your child's needs change. Schools must present parents with a copy of their rights at every meeting and upon request. It is also important to note that parents can invite anyone to the meeting they deem necessary, including outside therapists, tutors, and legal counsel.

A collaborative relationship with the school is essential to develop and implement an effective IEP or 504 Plan. This involves regular communication with teachers, special education staff, and administrators. It's important to approach these relationships with a spirit of partnership, working together to find the best strategies to support your child's learning and development. IEPs and 504 Plans are powerful tools in ensuring that your child with ADHD receives an education tailored to their unique needs. By understanding these plans and actively participating in their development, you play a crucial role in your child's educational journey, advocating for the accommodations and support they need to succeed.

ADVOCATING FOR YOUR CHILD'S NEEDS

As a parent of a child with ADHD, you take on the crucial role of being their advocate in the educational system. Advocacy goes beyond mere representation; it's about being a voice for your child, ensuring their needs and rights are upheld. This role is multifaceted and involves being well-informed, proactive, and collaborative.

Knowledge is power, and this is particularly true when advocating for a child with ADHD. Understanding ADHD and its impact on learning and behavior is fundamental. This knowledge helps you explain your child's needs to educators and advocate for appropriate accommodations. Stay updated on the latest research, treatment options, and educational strategies related to ADHD. This information empowers you to engage in informed discussions with educators and participate actively in decision-making processes.

Every child with ADHD is unique, and what works for one child may not work for another. It's vital to communicate your child's specific needs to their educators. Share insights about their strengths, challenges, and what has been effective or ineffective in the past. This information is invaluable for teachers in understanding and supporting your child in the classroom.

Advocacy also involves voicing concerns and making suggestions for your child's educational approach. This might include discussing potential classroom accommodations, behavior management strategies, or specific teaching methods that resonate with your child. Remember, your perspective as a parent is critical in shaping a supportive and effective educational experience for your child.

Effective advocacy is built on collaboration, not confrontation. Work alongside teachers, counselors, and administrators as partners in your child's education. Attend meetings prepared with observations and questions, and be open to suggestions from school personnel. Your goal is to create a supportive educational environment that recognizes and accommodates your child's ADHD, not to impose your views.

Lastly, as an advocate, you must be aware of your child's legal rights. Children with ADHD are entitled to certain protections and accommodations under federal laws like the Individuals with Disabilities Education Act (IDEA) and Section 504 of the Rehabilitation Act. Familiarize yourself with these laws to ensure your child's educational rights are recognized and fully upheld.

Advocating for your child's needs is an ongoing process that requires commitment, knowledge, and collaboration. It's about ensuring the educational system provides the support and accommodations necessary for your child to thrive. As their advocate, you are pivotal in navigating this journey, championing their needs, and celebrating their successes.

SECTION 2: EFFECTIVE LEARNING TECHNIQUES

In this section, we explore innovative and effective learning techniques specially designed for children with ADHD, moving beyond traditional education methods to embrace more dynamic, interactive, and personalized approaches. Tailored teaching strategies are at the forefront, emphasizing the need for engaging, hands-on learning experiences. These methods are not just about keeping children interested; they are crucial in resonating with their unique thinking patterns and high energy levels, enhancing their overall engagement and effectiveness in learning. Recognizing that every child with ADHD has a distinct journey, these strategies focus on customizing education to fit their needs and strengths.

We will also discuss the crucial role of incorporating regular breaks and physical activity into the learning routine and the innovative use of technology and educational apps. Breaks, especially those involving physical activity, are more than just pauses in the day; they are essential for managing energy levels and boosting concentration. Alongside this, the digital age offers many technological tools and apps that can greatly aid in organizing, engaging, and facilitating learning for children with ADHD. This segment provides practical advice on how to effectively integrate these elements into both school and home environments, transforming the challenges of ADHD into opportunities for success and growth in your child's educational journey.

TAILORED TEACHING STRATEGIES

When it comes to educating children with ADHD, the traditional *'one-size-fits-all'* teaching approach often falls short. These children typically thrive in environments where the learning methods are as dynamic and varied as their needs and strengths. Tailored teaching strategies, therefore, become essential in facilitating their educational journey. These strategies focus on customization to fit the unique learning styles of each child with ADHD.

Interactive and hands-on learning is a cornerstone of this approach. Unlike traditional methods that primarily rely on passive learning, interactive learning encourages active participation from students. It involves activities where children can physically engage with the material, such as through experiments, building projects, or role-playing scenarios. This type of learning helps maintain their interest and caters to their kinesthetic learning preferences, where they learn best by doing.

Incorporating movement and activity into lessons is another key strategy. Children with ADHD often find it challenging to sit still for prolonged periods, which can hinder their ability to focus and absorb information. Integrating movement into the learning process can help these students channel their energy positively. This could be as simple as allowing them to stand while working, having stretch breaks, or including activities that involve moving around the classroom. These small adjustments can significantly affect their ability to concentrate and participate in lessons.

Finally, tapping into the interests of children with ADHD can be a powerful tool in engaging their attention. When lessons incorporate topics or themes they are passionate about, their natural curiosity and enthusiasm are ignited. This could involve using their favorite books, characters, or hobbies as contexts for learning. For instance, a math lesson can be built around a child's interest in space exploration, or a language arts assignment can be centered on a sport they love. This makes learning more enjoyable and demonstrates to the child that their interests are valued and understood.

By embracing these tailored teaching strategies, we can create a learning environment that is not only more accommodating and effective for children with ADHD but also one that celebrates and leverages their unique perspectives and abilities.

THE IMPORTANCE OF BREAKS AND PHYSICAL ACTIVITY

For children with ADHD, the traditional model of long, uninterrupted periods of classroom learning can be particularly challenging. Their natural disposition towards higher energy levels and the need for frequent mental rest make incorporating regular breaks and physical activity beneficial and essential. These elements play a critical role in managing their energy and enhancing their ability to concentrate, ultimately positively impacting their overall academic experience.

Regular breaks during the school day provide necessary mental respite for children with ADHD. These pauses are vital in preventing cognitive overload, a common issue for these children who may struggle with sustained attention. Short, structured breaks - ranging from a brief moment of stretching to a few minutes of walking or quiet time - allow these students to reset their focus and return to their tasks with renewed concentration. This strategy acknowledges and accommodates their need for periodic disengagement from the continuous cognitive effort, thereby aiding in maintaining a more consistent level of productivity throughout the day.

Physical activity is equally important and serves multiple purposes for children with ADHD. Engaging in physical exercises or movement-based activities not only helps in expending excess energy but also aids in boosting brain function. Activities such as a quick game, a walk outside, or simple classroom exercises can significantly enhance their cognitive abilities. Physical activity has been shown to increase alertness and improve mood, conducive to better learning. Additionally, it can serve as a positive reinforcement, motivating children to engage with their learning tasks.

UTILIZING TECHNOLOGY AND APPS FOR LEARNING

In today's digital era, technology is a formidable ally in educating children with ADHD. The plethora of apps and digital tools available today are not just supplementary; they are revolutionizing how these children learn, interact with, and process information. These technologies enhance focus, improve organization, and facilitate a more engaging learning experience, making them invaluable assets for children with ADHD.

One of the primary advantages of using technology in education for children with ADHD is its ability to hold their attention in ways traditional methods may not. Interactive and visually appealing apps can transform learning into an engaging experience, capturing their interest and increasing their focus and retention of information. Educational games, for instance, can turn challenging subjects into fun activities. Similarly, storytelling apps can bring narratives to life, aiding in better comprehension and recall.

Organization is another area where technology can be incredibly beneficial for children with ADHD. Many struggle with executive functions, such as organizing tasks or managing time effectively. Various apps are designed to help, offering features like digital planners, reminder systems, and step-by-step task breakdowns. These tools can help children structure their day, keep track of assignments and deadlines, and develop a sense of independence and competence in managing their responsibilities.

Furthermore, technology can provide personalized learning experiences. Adaptive learning apps can tailor the difficulty and type of content based on the child's responses, ensuring that the material is neither easy nor hard. This customization is crucial for keeping children with ADHD challenged but not overwhelmed, fostering an environment conducive to learning at their own pace and ability level.

Incorporating technology and apps into a child's learning process requires mindful selection and moderation. It's important to choose reputable, age-appropriate apps that are aligned with educational goals. Parents and educators should also monitor the usage to ensure that screen time is balanced and does not replace other essential learning and developmental activities. Embracing technology in education offers a modern, flexible, and effective approach to learning for children with ADHD. When used thoughtfully, these digital tools can significantly enhance the educational experience, providing a stimulating and supportive environment that caters to their unique learning needs.

SECTION 3: OVERCOMING ACADEMIC HURDLES

Now, we turn our attention to overcoming the academic hurdles that children with ADHD often encounter. This part of the chapter addresses the common academic challenges these children face, including issues with focus, organization, and managing the complexities of schoolwork. We understand that these challenges can be daunting, but they can be navigated successfully with the right strategies and support. We aim to provide parents with practical and effective tools to help their children cope with these challenges and thrive academically.

Here, we will delve into the development of crucial study skills and homework strategies that are tailored to the unique needs of children with ADHD. These strategies foster a sense of control and competence in managing school tasks. Additionally, we will tackle the often-overlooked issue of test anxiety and performance pressure, which can be particularly intense for these children.

We'll explore techniques to manage this anxiety, preparing your child to face tests and assessments confidently and resiliently. By equipping parents with this knowledge, we aim to empower them to guide their children through the academic landscape with greater ease and effectiveness, paving the way for their long-term educational success.

ADDRESSING COMMON ACADEMIC CHALLENGES

Children with ADHD frequently encounter a unique set of academic challenges that can significantly impact their educational journey. Among the most common are difficulties with executive functions, encompassing skills such as organization, time management, and task initiation. These challenges can create significant barriers to learning and academic success without appropriate intervention. However, these obstacles can be overcome with early identification and targeted strategies, paving the way for a more positive and productive educational experience.

Organization is a primary area of difficulty for many children with ADHD. This manifests in various ways, from keeping track of school materials to organizing thoughts for writing assignments or breaking down large projects into manageable parts. Specific strategies, such as using color-coded systems for different subjects, employing graphic organizers for writing, or maintaining a clear, structured routine, can greatly assist in reducing overwhelm and helping children stay on track.

Time management is another critical executive function with which children with ADHD often struggle. Understanding how long tasks will take and planning accordingly can be daunting for these children. Teaching them to use planners or digital calendars, setting task timers, and creating visual schedules are effective ways to develop time management skills. Breaking tasks into smaller steps with clear deadlines can help them manage their workload better.

In addition to these executive function challenges, children with ADHD often face issues with focus and attention, impulsive behaviors in the classroom, slow processing speed, and social skills challenges. These can lead to inconsistent academic performance, memory, reading, and writing difficulties. Strategies to address these include breaking tasks into shorter segments, setting clear classroom rules, allowing extra time for tests, incorporating social skills training, and using repetition and mnemonic devices to aid memory.

Recognizing that these challenges are not due to a lack of effort or motivation is crucial. Children with ADHD may need more guidance and structure than their peers to develop these skills. Parents and educators play a vital role in providing this support, teaching these skills, providing consistent reinforcement, and offering opportunities to practice them in various settings. Early intervention is key in addressing these challenges, helping to alleviate immediate academic struggles and setting the foundation for long-term success. This proactive approach empowers children with ADHD to develop the skills and strategies to navigate their academic journey confidently and resiliently.

STUDY SKILLS AND HOMEWORK STRATEGIES

For children with ADHD, mastering study skills and homework strategies is not just about completing assignments; it's about cultivating habits and techniques that enhance learning and foster a sense of achievement. Creating a structured approach to studying and homework can significantly improve the educational experience for these children. This involves implementing routines, using visual aids, and tailoring study techniques to align with their individual learning styles.

Structured routines play a pivotal role in helping children with ADHD to focus and manage their tasks effectively. A consistent routine demystifies what is expected and reduces anxiety and the likelihood of becoming overwhelmed. This could mean having a set time and quiet place for homework each day, with all necessary materials readily available. Such predictability in their schedule aids in transitioning more smoothly into study mode and maintaining focus throughout the session.

Visual aids are another valuable tool in enhancing organization and comprehension. For many children with ADHD, visual cues are more effective than verbal instructions. Using color-coded folders or notebooks for different subjects, visual planners showing weekly or monthly tasks, and checklists for daily assignments can help them keep track of their work and progress. These aids are constant reminders of what needs to be done, reducing the chances of forgetting tasks or deadlines.

Tailoring study techniques to your child's learning style is an important consideration. Children with ADHD often have unique ways of processing information, and recognizing this can guide the selection of effective study methods. For instance, incorporating physical activities or hands-on experiments can enhance understanding and retention if your child is a kinesthetic learner. For auditory learners, discussing the material aloud or using educational videos or podcasts might be more effective. Similarly, using diagrams, mind maps, or flashcards can benefit visual learners.

Additionally, breaking down larger assignments into smaller, manageable tasks can help prevent feelings of being overwhelmed. This approach and short breaks can keep motivation and energy levels steady. Encouraging self-reflection on what strategies work best and gradually fostering independence in managing their study and homework routines can also contribute significantly to their academic growth.

By focusing on developing these study and homework strategies, parents and educators can provide children with ADHD with the tools and confidence they need to succeed academically. These strategies aid in completing immediate tasks and instill valuable skills throughout their educational journey and into adulthood.

Test anxiety and performance pressure are common and often heightened challenges for children with ADHD. The high-stakes environment of tests and exams can exacerbate their symptoms, leading to increased stress and, consequently, a hindrance in their ability to showcase their true capabilities. However, with the right strategies and preparations, this anxiety can be managed effectively, allowing these children to approach tests more confidently and calmly.

One of the key strategies in managing test anxiety is teaching children relaxation techniques. Deep breathing exercises, progressive muscle relaxation, or guided imagery can reduce stress. These methods help calm the mind and body, making it easier for children to focus. Parents and educators can teach these techniques and encourage children to practice them regularly, not just during test situations but as part of their daily routine. This regular practice can make it easier for children to access these techniques when needed.

Preparation is another critical element in managing test anxiety. This doesn't just mean studying the material well in advance, although that is certainly important. It also involves familiarizing the child with the test format, practicing under similar conditions, and developing a plan for tackling the test. For example, they can practice answering questions within a set time limit or write mock tests to build familiarity and confidence. Helping children develop a structured study plan that breaks down the material into manageable sections can also reduce feeling overwhelmed.

Having supportive strategies in place during tests is also essential. This can include allowing breaks during the test, providing a quiet space to reduce distractions, or permitting using stress-relief tools like fidget spinners or stress balls. Additionally, discussing possible accommodations with the child's teacher, such as extended time or different testing environments, can be beneficial. It's important for the child to know that these supports are in place, as this knowledge alone can help reduce anxiety. In managing test anxiety and performance pressure, the goal is to equip children with ADHD with the skills and strategies they need to navigate these high-pressure situations. By doing so, we can help them demonstrate their true abilities and knowledge in a test setting, thereby improving their academic experience and outcomes.

Navigating and mastering the educational challenges faced by children with ADHD is a multifaceted journey. The strategies and insights, from tailored teaching methods to managing test anxiety, are designed to create a supportive and effective learning environment. However, our goal extends beyond academic success. It is equally important to focus on fostering independence in our children with ADHD. This journey toward independence is not just about academic achievements; it's about equipping them with the skills and confidence to navigate the world on their own terms.

While mastering the academic hurdles is undeniably important, it is equally essential to prepare our children for the broader challenges of life. We'll explore practical steps and strategies to help them build independence in their academic pursuits and everyday life scenarios, setting the stage for their long-term success and personal growth.

CHAPTER EIGHT

FOSTERING INDEPENDENCE AND RESPONSIBILITY

*M*eet Erica, a vivacious 13-year-old diagnosed with ADHD. Her energy seems limitless, her ideas a constant whirlwind, and her creativity shines in every aspect of her life. But Erica's journey hasn't been without its challenges. As a younger child, she often struggled with organization, forgetfulness, and the myriad of small tasks that make up daily life. Her parents, though supportive, were frequently fraught with concerns about her future. How would Erica, with her scatter-brained tendencies and impulsiveness, navigate the complexities of growing up?

Fast forward to the present, and you'll find a remarkably different picture. Erica isn't just coping; she's thriving. She excels in schoolwork, a feat that once seemed a distant dream. But perhaps most impressively, Erica has channeled her boundless energy into a successful venture – a small online business where she sells her handcrafted jewelry. This isn't just a hobby; it's a testament to her growing sense of responsibility, her burgeoning independence, and her ability to channel her ADHD traits into productive, fulfilling endeavors.

How did this transformation occur? Was it a sudden change or a gradual evolution? The truth lies somewhere in between. Erica's journey to independence and responsibility was paved with patience, understanding, and strategic interventions. It's a journey that many parents of children with ADHD aspire to navigate successfully.

In this chapter, we discuss this transformative process in depth, offering a comprehensive guide for parents who face similar challenges and harbor similar hopes for their children. You'll discover practical strategies, real-life anecdotes, and expert advice tailored to help your child harness their unique strengths, overcome their struggles, and journey towards a future brimming with potential.

From setting age-appropriate expectations to nurturing life skills and preparing for adulthood, this chapter will equip you with the tools and insights necessary to support your child's path to independence and responsibility. Erica's story isn't just one of personal achievement; it's a blueprint for success that can inspire and guide parents and children alike in the ADHD community. Let's explore this journey together, learning and growing every step of the way.

SECTION 1: AGE-APPROPRIATE EXPECTATIONS

Fostering independence in a child with ADHD is not about imposing our expectations but understanding and nurturing their unique journey. This section is designed to guide you, as a parent, in setting realistic and achievable goals for your child's autonomy, tailored to their individual developmental stage and abilities. We'll explore how to tailor expectations appropriately, recognizing the significance of each small step your child takes toward autonomy.

The emphasis here is on progress, not perfection, and on building a sense of accomplishment in your child. Through a stepwise approach, we guide you in gradually introducing responsibilities, helping your child build confidence and capability in managing their tasks. Additionally, we stress the importance of celebrating milestones, big and small, reinforcing the positive strides your child makes.

As you navigate this section, remember the individuality of your child's journey toward independence and your support's pivotal role in their development. This is about laying a foundation for growth, step by step, aligning with your child's unique strengths and challenges.

SETTING REALISTIC GOALS FOR AUTONOMY

In guiding children with ADHD towards autonomy, setting realistic and age-appropriate goals is a fundamental step. This approach respects their unique developmental stage and capabilities, ensuring the goals are challenging yet achievable, which is key to building their confidence and independence. Each child's developmental journey is unique, especially for those with ADHD.

Understanding where your child stands regarding their cognitive, emotional, and physical development is crucial. Young children, for example, are just learning to manage basic tasks and need goals that align with these early developmental stages.

Young Children

Self-Care: Encourage your young child to do simple self-care tasks, such as dressing, brushing their teeth, or combing their hair. You might need to break these tasks into smaller steps first and patiently guide them through each step.

Organizing and Tidying Up: Teach them to organize their toys and belongings. Use clear and simple storage systems, and label shelves or bins with pictures to make it easier for them to remember where things go.

Following Simple Routines: Establish simple morning and bedtime routines. Visual schedules can be very helpful, allowing them to see what tasks need to be done and in what order.

School-Age Children

Homework Management: Start introducing responsibilities related to school, such as completing homework independently or packing their school bag. Use tools like planners or checklists to help them keep track of assignments and deadlines.

Household Chores: Assign age-appropriate chores, such as setting the table, feeding a pet, or helping with meal preparation. This teaches responsibility and instills a sense of belonging and contribution to the family.

Time Management: Introduce concepts like time management through timers or alarms, especially for activities children with ADHD might lose track of time on, like playing or watching TV.

Pre-Teens and Teenagers

Advanced School Responsibilities: Encourage them to take on more complex school-related tasks, like managing multiple assignments, participating in extracurricular activities, or preparing for exams.

Financial Management: Teach them about managing money by giving them a small allowance. Guide them in budgeting, saving for something they want, and making thoughtful spending decisions.

Self-Advocacy: Encourage them to express their needs, especially in school settings. Teach them to ask for help and communicate effectively with teachers and peers.

It's important to remember that the goal isn't to achieve perfection but to make continuous progress. Children with ADHD may face more challenges in achieving these milestones, and it's essential to recognize and celebrate each small achievement. This approach builds their self-esteem and reinforces their ability to overcome new challenges. Be flexible and ready to adjust goals based on your child's progress and response. What works for one child may not work for another, even within the same family. Regularly assess and modify goals to ensure they remain challenging yet attainable, keeping in mind the ultimate aim of fostering independence in your child.

THE STEP-WISE APPROACH TO RESPONSIBILITY

For children, especially those with ADHD, developing a sense of responsibility is a gradual process. It requires patience, understanding, and a strategic approach. The stepwise method of introducing and building responsibilities is highly effective, allowing children to gain confidence and skills progressively.

Begin by assigning simple, manageable tasks your child can easily comprehend and execute. These tasks should be age-appropriate and can be completed with minimal assistance. Young children can work on tasks like putting toys away after playing, placing dirty clothes in the laundry basket, or helping to water plants. These activities are straightforward and establish the foundational concept of responsibility. For older children, you can introduce slightly more complex tasks such as helping to set the table for meals, sorting and folding their laundry, or caring for a family pet.

Gradually introduce more challenging ones once your child becomes comfortable and consistent with simpler tasks. This progression should be based on their ability to manage previous tasks successfully. For instance, if your child has mastered setting the table, the next step could be helping to prepare simple dishes or snacks. If they've successfully cared for a pet, they can take on additional responsibilities like walking the dog or cleaning its living space. Finally, make sure you allow them to have a say in what new responsibilities they would like to take on. This sense of choice can be very empowering and motivating.

Always provide positive reinforcement and constructive feedback. Praise their efforts and accomplishments, no matter how small. This encouragement will bolster their confidence and motivation. As we mentioned, consider a reward system for consistently completing responsibilities, but ensure the rewards are reasonable and not overly extravagant. The focus should be on intrinsic motivation rather than external rewards.

Be prepared to adapt to the responsibilities based on your child's responses and challenges. If a task seems too overwhelming, break it down into smaller, more manageable steps or replace it with a more suitable task. Maintain an open line of communication with your child. Ask them how they feel about their responsibilities and what challenges they might be facing. This dialogue is crucial for understanding their perspective and making necessary adjustments.

The stepwise approach to responsibility is a journey of gradual progression, consistent reinforcement, and adaptability. It is designed to build not just a sense of responsibility in children with ADHD but also to foster their self-esteem, independence, and a positive attitude towards challenges and accomplishments.

CELEBRATING MILESTONE AND ACHIEVEMENTS

Positive reinforcement is a powerful tool, especially for children with ADHD who may struggle with self-esteem and motivation. Celebrating milestones and achievements, big or small, acknowledges their effort and progress, fostering a sense of accomplishment and pride.

Milestones can vary significantly from child to child, depending on their age, abilities, and the challenges they face due to ADHD. These can range from completing homework without reminders and maintaining an organized room to larger accomplishments like achieving good grades or participating in extracurricular activities. The key is to recognize the effort rather than just the outcome.

Here are some ways to celebrate milestones:

Verbal Praise: Simple words of encouragement and acknowledgment can be incredibly uplifting. Phrases like *"I'm proud of you for completing your homework on time"* or *"You did a great job organizing your room"* can make a huge difference.

Reward Systems: Implement a reward system where your child earns points or tokens for completing tasks or achieving goals. These can be exchanged for small rewards, such as extra screen time, a special outing, or a small gift.

Certificate or Chart: Create a visual representation of their achievements, like a certificate of achievement or a progress chart displayed in a common area of the home. This celebrates their successes and visually reminds them of their progress.

Family Celebrations: Mark significant achievements with a family celebration. This could be a special meal, a family game night, or an outing. This approach reinforces the idea that their achievements are important to the family.

Personalized Rewards: Tailor rewards to your child's interests and passions. For example, if your child loves art, reward them with new art supplies or visit an art museum.

Involving Them in the Planning: For bigger achievements, involve your child in planning the celebration. This gives them a sense of control and acknowledges their maturity.

The impact of celebrating achievements in children with ADHD is multifaceted and profoundly beneficial. Regular recognition and positive reinforcement play a critical role in building self-confidence. Children with ADHD often encounter repeated criticisms, making it essential to bolster their self-esteem through positive acknowledgments of their efforts and accomplishments. Moreover, celebrating these achievements has a significant effect on their motivation. When children see their efforts being recognized, they are more likely to repeat those behaviors, creating a positive feedback loop. This cycle motivates them to take on new challenges and responsibilities and helps ingrain those positive behaviors.

Additionally, celebrating achievements together can greatly strengthen the parent-child bond. It sends a clear message to the child that their parents are not just observers but active and supportive participants in their journey. This shared joy and pride in accomplishments demonstrate to the child that their efforts are valued and noticed, fostering a deeper connection and understanding within the family unit.

Finally, recognizing achievements effectively teaches children the value of setting and working towards goals. This skill is invaluable as they grow and face more complex life challenges. Understanding the process of setting a goal, working towards it, and celebrating the achievement lays a strong foundation for future success in various aspects of life. It instills a sense of purpose and direction, which is especially crucial for children with ADHD, who may struggle with focusing and seeing tasks to completion. In essence, celebrating achievements is not just about acknowledging success but equipping children with ADHD with the tools and confidence they need to navigate life's challenges. Always remember, what might seem like a small step for others can be a giant leap for a child with ADHD.

SECTION 2: LIFE SKILLS TRAINING

This section focuses on the practical aspects of nurturing independence in children with ADHD. Here, we delve into the essential skills that pave the way for self-sufficiency and lay the groundwork for long-term personal growth and success. We begin by exploring the different life skills appropriate for various age groups. From basic self-care for younger children to more complex tasks like financial management for teenagers, this section provides a roadmap for gradually equipping your child with the skills they need at each stage of their development.

In addition to practical skills, we emphasize the importance of encouraging personal growth and ambition. It's about helping your child find their passions and interests and supporting them in setting and pursuing their goals. Lastly, we address a crucial aspect of growing up with ADHD: financial literacy. This section aims to empower your child with the knowledge and confidence to manage finances responsibly, an essential skill for their journey into adulthood.

As you navigate this section, remember that teaching life skills to a child with ADHD is as much about patience and understanding as the skills themselves. It's about preparing your child for today's challenges and tomorrow's opportunities.

DAILY LIVING SKILLS FOR DIFFERENT AGE GROUPS

Developing daily living skills is crucial for children with ADHD, as it fosters independence and instills a sense of accomplishment and self-worth. The key is gradually and appropriately introducing these skills based on the child's age and individual capabilities.

Skills for Younger Children (Ages 4-7)

Basic Hygiene: Teach them the importance of daily personal hygiene routines such as brushing teeth, bathing, and washing hands. Use visual aids like charts or fun videos to engage the learning process.

Tidying Up: Encourage them to keep their room and play area organized. Start by showing them how to put toys away after playtime and gradually introduce them to tasks like making their bed.

Dressing Themselves: Help them learn how to choose appropriate clothes for the weather and dress themselves. You can make this fun by turning it into a game or challenge.

Simple Food Preparation: Introduce them to basic food preparation like spreading butter on bread or pouring cereal and milk. Always supervise and ensure safety measures are in place.

Skills for Pre-Teens (Ages 8-12)

Cooking Simple Meals: Teach them to prepare simple meals like sandwiches, salads, or basic pasta. Start with recipes that don't require sharp knives or hot stoves, gradually progressing to more complex tasks.

Managing Schedules: Help them learn to manage their time effectively. Introduce them to tools like planners or digital calendars. Encourage them to write down important dates like project deadlines or extracurricular activities.

Basic Laundry Tasks: Show them how to sort clothes, use the washing machine, and fold clean laundry. Start with easy tasks like pairing socks and work up to operating the washer and dryer with supervision.

Responsibility for Personal Belongings: Teach them to take care of their personal belongings, like organizing their school bag, keeping track of their library books, or taking care of their electronics.

Skills for Teenagers (Ages 13-18)

Advanced Cooking: Encourage them to try more complex recipes, including using the stove and oven. Focus on teaching them to prepare healthy, balanced meals.

Doing Laundry: At this stage, they should be able to handle their laundry independently, including understanding laundry symbols and choosing the right wash settings.

Basic Home Repairs: Teach them simple home repair tasks like unclogging a drain, changing a lightbulb, or fixing a leaky faucet. These skills are invaluable for when they live on their own.

Budgeting and Financial Management: Introduce budgeting, saving, and responsible spending concepts. Give them opportunities to manage small amounts of money or use educational apps to teach financial literacy.

Planning and Organizing: Encourage them to plan and organize more complex activities, like a school project, a trip, or a weekly schedule. This fosters time management and prioritization skills.

By teaching these skills tailored to each age group, parents can significantly aid their children with ADHD in becoming more self-reliant and prepared for the challenges of adulthood. Remember, patience and consistent reinforcement are key, as children with ADHD may need more time and practice to master these skills.

ENCOURAGING PERSONAL GROWTH AND AMBITION

Fostering personal growth and ambition in children with ADHD involves a delicate balance of guidance and freedom. This journey is about setting goals and understanding and nurturing your child's unique interests and aspirations. Doing so, you help them develop a sense of self-worth and a desire to pursue their dreams.

The first step in encouraging personal growth is understanding what excites and truly motivates your child. This can be a dynamic process, as interests may evolve over time. Engage in open-ended conversations, observe their play patterns, and note what subjects or activities draw their attention. Remember, their passions might differ from your expectations or the typical interests of their age group, and that's perfectly okay.

Once you grasp your child's interests, guide them in setting achievable goals. These goals should be specific, measurable, attainable, relevant, and time-bound (SMART). For a child fascinated by cooking, a goal might be to learn to prepare a new dish each month. If they are interested in sports, perhaps aiming to improve a specific skill or achieve a new personal best can be a goal. Ensure that these goals are challenging yet attainable to maintain motivation and interest.

After setting goals, the next step is to create a plan to achieve them. This roadmap should include clear, small steps and consider any potential obstacles, especially those unique to ADHD, like difficulty maintaining focus. For instance, if the goal is to learn a musical instrument, the plan might include regular practice sessions, each with a specific focus, and breaks to manage attention span effectively.

Children with ADHD often benefit from visual aids and organizational tools. Consider using planners, charts, or apps to help your child track their progress. Breaking tasks into smaller, manageable parts can also be helpful. Regular check-ins to review progress and adjust goals as needed can keep your child engaged and focused.

Your role as a parent is to provide a supportive and encouraging environment. Celebrate successes, no matter how small, and offer constructive feedback when things are unplanned. Teach them that setbacks are part of the learning process and not a reflection of their worth or abilities. External support like mentors, tutors, or clubs can provide additional guidance and encouragement. Look for community resources, after-school programs, or online forums where your child can connect with others who share their interests.

Encourage your child to think beyond immediate goals and consider their long-term aspirations. This broader perspective helps them see the connection between their interests and future possibilities. For instance, a child interested in building models might be encouraged to explore careers in engineering or architecture.

Finally, be prepared to embrace changes. As your child grows and explores, their interests and goals might shift. This is a natural part of personal growth. The key is to remain supportive and adaptive, helping them confidently navigate these changes. By encouraging personal growth and ambition in your child with ADHD, you're not only helping them develop specific skills or achieve certain goals. You're also instilling a lifelong love for learning, a sense of purpose, and the confidence to pursue their dreams, no matter where they lead.

FINANCIAL LITERACY FOR YOUNG ADULTS WITH ADHD

Financial literacy is an essential life skill for young adults. The unique challenges children with ADHD face, such as impulsivity and difficulty in planning, make it crucial to cultivate good financial habits early on. This section outlines strategies to help your child understand and manage money effectively.

Understanding the Basics of Money Management: Start with the fundamentals of money. Explain the value of money and how it is earned. Discuss the difference between needs and wants and the importance of making informed spending choices. Integrate simple examples to make these concepts relatable, like comparing the cost of items your child is familiar with.

Budgeting Basics: Introduce the concept of budgeting. Create a simple budget with your child, allocating funds for savings, expenses, and leisure. Use visual aids like charts or budgeting apps designed for young people. This hands-on experience makes the process more engaging and understandable.

The Art of Saving: Teach the importance of saving. Encourage your child to set a savings goal, such as buying a desired item or saving for a special event. Open a savings account in their name and guide them on how to deposit money into it. Discuss the concept of interest and how savings grow over time.

Using Prepaid Credit Cards: Prepaid credit cards can be an excellent tool for learning financial responsibility. They allow teens to make purchases while limiting the risk of overspending. Teach them to track their spending, balance, and reload the card. This experience can provide a sense of independence and a practical understanding of credit card usage.

Smart Spending Habits: Discuss strategies for responsible spending. Teach your child to compare prices, look for discounts, and understand the difference between high-quality and expensive items. Encourage them to think twice before making impulse purchases and to prioritize their spending based on their budget.

Dealing with Mistakes: Mistakes are inevitable and can be valuable learning experiences. If your child overspends or makes a poor financial decision, use this to discuss what went wrong and how to make better choices in the future. Emphasize that making mistakes is part of learning how to manage money effectively.

Planning for the Future: Talk about long-term financial planning, including saving for college, a car, or other significant future expenses. Introduce the concept of investments and how they can be a part of future financial planning. This helps in instilling a sense of future orientation and goal setting.

Financial literacy is a critical skill for independence and success in adulthood. For young adults with ADHD, mastering these skills can be particularly empowering. By taking a step-by-step approach and using practical tools like prepaid credit cards, you can help your child build a strong foundation in financial management. This foundation will serve them in their immediate future and pave the way for responsible financial decisions in their adult life.

SECTION 3: PREPARING FOR ADULTHOOD

In this chapter, we address the critical phase of transitioning from childhood to adulthood for children with ADHD. This stage is not just about building upon previously learned skills; it's about equipping your child for adult life's broader challenges and opportunities. This section guides you through the nuances of parenting during the teenage years—a time when ADHD can present unique challenges. We'll explore strategies to balance offering support and allowing independence, ensuring your child feels empowered to make their own decisions. We also discuss the specific challenges that adolescents with ADHD may face. This includes managing impulsivity, maintaining focus, and navigating social relationships.

Understanding these challenges is key to providing the right support and guidance. Finally, we delve into planning for independent living. This involves conversations about further education, career paths, and life skills necessary for living independently. We'll provide insights into helping your child explore various options and make informed decisions about their future.

As you read this section, remember that preparing for adulthood is a gradual process that requires patience, empathy, and encouragement. It's about giving your child the tools and confidence to enter adulthood with a sense of readiness and optimism.

PARENTING TIPS FOR THE TEENAGE YEARS

Navigating the teenage years with a child who has ADHD can be a complex and challenging journey. As a parent, it's crucial to balance guiding your teen and allowing them the freedom to make their own decisions. This balance is not just about maintaining peace at home; it's about fostering independence and preparing your teen for adulthood.

Here are some key strategies and tips to help you through these pivotal years:

Open and Honest Communication: Establish a relationship where your teen feels comfortable sharing their thoughts and feelings with you. Encourage open dialogue and listen actively. Remember, communication is not just about speaking; it's equally about listening. Validate their feelings and experiences, even if you don't always agree with them.

Setting Clear Expectations: Teens with ADHD often benefit from clear and consistent expectations. This includes rules around curfews, homework, chores, and social activities. Be clear about the consequences of not meeting these expectations, and ensure they are fair and consistent.

Encouraging Independence: Gradually give your teen more responsibility. This could be in the form of more significant household chores, managing their own schedules, or making decisions about their extracurricular activities. The goal is to help them feel capable and independent

Managing ADHD Symptoms: Continue to work with your teen on strategies to manage ADHD symptoms. This might include organizing their space, using planners or digital tools for time management, and breaking tasks into smaller, manageable steps.

Promoting Self-Awareness: Help your teen recognize their strengths and challenges. Encourage them to recognize how ADHD affects them personally and how to advocate for themselves, especially in educational settings.

Building Self-Esteem: Focus on your teen's strengths and accomplishments. Celebrate their successes, no matter how small. Positive reinforcement can boost their self-esteem and motivation.

Teaching Decision-Making skills: Guide your teen in making decisions by discussing potential outcomes and encouraging them to weigh the pros and cons. This practice helps them develop critical thinking and problem-solving skills.

Handling Mistakes: Teach your teen that making mistakes is a part of learning and growing. Help them understand how to learn from these mistakes and move forward without dwelling on them.

Prioritizing Mental Health: Be attentive to your teen's mental health. Adolescents with ADHD are at a higher risk for anxiety and depression. Encourage open conversations about mental health and seek professional help if needed.

Maintaining a Supportive Environment: Create a supportive home environment that understands your teen's ADHD. This includes being patient, avoiding criticism for ADHD-related difficulties, and providing unconditional love and support.

Staying Informed and Involved: Stay informed about ADHD and how it affects teenagers. Be involved in their education and collaborate with teachers and counselors to ensure your teen has the support they need at school.

Planning for the Furure: Start conversations about life after high school. Discuss different options, whether it's college, vocational training, or entering the workforce. Help them explore their interests and find paths that align with their strengths and skills.

By implementing these strategies, you can help your teen with ADHD navigate the challenges of adolescence while fostering a sense of independence and responsibility. Remember, each teen is unique, and what works for one may not work for another. The key is patience, understanding, and a willingness to adapt as your child grows and changes.

CHALLENGES OF ADHD DURING ADOLESCENCE

Adolescence is a transformative period marked by significant physical, emotional, and social changes. For children with ADHD, these changes often intensify the challenges they face. Understanding and addressing these specific challenges is crucial for successfully helping your child navigate these formative years.

During adolescence, individuals with ADHD may exhibit increased impulsivity and a propensity for risk-taking behaviors. This can manifest in various ways, from experimenting with substances to engaging in unsafe driving practices. It's important to have open discussions about these risks. Create a safe space for your child to talk about peer pressure and help them develop strategies to make safer choices. Encourage activities that channel their energy positively, like sports or creative arts.

The academic and social demands of adolescence can exacerbate focus issues in children with ADHD. They struggle more with organizing tasks, managing time, and maintaining attention in class. Work with your child's teachers to develop a supportive educational plan. Tools like planners, timers, and breaks during study sessions can help manage these tasks. Encourage your child to use technology responsibly, as it can be both a tool and a distraction.

Social interactions become more complex in adolescence, and children with ADHD may feel out of step with their peers. They might have difficulty interpreting social cues or may act in ways that are seen as inappropriate. If necessary, encourage your child to engage in social skills training or therapy. Role-playing common social scenarios at home can also be beneficial. Foster an environment where they feel comfortable discussing their social experiences and concerns.

Adolescents with ADHD often experience heightened emotions and may struggle with mood swings or frustration. These emotional regulation difficulties can lead to conflicts at home and school. Teach your child techniques to manage emotions, like deep breathing or mindfulness. Consistent routines and clear expectations at home can also provide a sense of stability.

The increased academic workload in adolescence can be overwhelming for children with ADHD. They might struggle with complex and longer assignments, leading to feelings of inadequacy or anxiety. Collaborate with educators to provide appropriate accommodations, such as extended time for tests or assignments.

Help your child break down tasks into smaller, manageable steps and celebrate their efforts and progress.

As they become more aware of their differences, adolescents with ADHD may struggle with self-esteem. It's important to emphasize their strengths and unique talents. Encourage pursuits where they can experience success and feel competent. Regular, positive feedback can help build their self-worth.

Thinking about the future can be daunting for adolescents with ADHD. They may struggle with decision-making or fear they won't be able to meet expectations. Engage in open conversations about their aspirations and concerns. Help them explore career paths or further education options that align with their strengths and interests.

Navigating adolescence with ADHD involves understanding and addressing these unique challenges. Through patience, open communication, and tailored strategies, you can empower your child to manage their ADHD symptoms effectively and thrive during these crucial years. Remember, every adolescent's journey is different, and what works for one child may not work for another. The key is to stay adaptive, supportive, and encouraging throughout this journey.

PLANNING FOR INDEPENDENT LIVING

As your child grows older, it becomes increasingly important to plan for their transition into adulthood. This phase involves nurturing their independence and guiding them in making significant life decisions about education, careers, and living arrangements. Start by having open and honest discussions about their aspirations and concerns regarding the future. Encourage your child to express their thoughts about what they want to do after high school. These conversations should be ongoing, evolving as your child's interests and abilities develop.

Exploring different educational paths is crucial in planning for your child's future. College is often seen as the traditional route, but it's not the only option available. Vocational training, community colleges, or specialized programs designed for individuals with ADHD can also be excellent choices. It's important to discuss the pros and cons of each option and consider visiting campuses or training centers together to get a real feel for what they offer.

Regarding career exploration, it's beneficial to help your child identify their strengths, interests, and values as they relate to potential careers. Utilizing resources such as career assessments or counseling can provide valuable insights.

Encourage your child to participate in job shadowing or internships in areas that pique their interest. It's essential to remember that it's perfectly okay for their career path to be non-linear or unconventional.

Working together with your child to develop a realistic and achievable plan is a key part of this journey. This plan should include short-term goals, like completing a specific course, and long-term objectives, such as gaining employment in a chosen field. Break these goals into smaller, manageable steps to make them more attainable. For instance, if the goal is to live independently, you might start by having your child consistently manage a specific household task.

Identifying the support and resources your child will need to achieve these goals is important. This could include tutoring, therapy, mentoring, or financial planning assistance. If further education or training is part of the plan, focus on developing the skills needed to succeed in that environment, such as time management, study skills, and self-advocacy. Develop essential skills such as resume writing, interviewing techniques, and workplace etiquette for employment readiness. Many communities offer programs specifically designed to help individuals with ADHD develop these skills.

Exploring various living arrangements with your child is crucial when planning for independent living. This exploration includes discussing options such as staying at home, living in a college dormitory, or renting an apartment. It's important to consider the kind of accommodations or support your child might need in each scenario. For instance, while living at home may provide a familiar environment, living in a dorm or an apartment might offer more independence and require greater self-management skills. Alongside these considerations, establishing safety nets and backup plans is equally important.

Life is unpredictable, and being prepared for challenges is wise. For example, if your child finds living independently more challenging than anticipated, having a plan for additional support or a temporary return home can provide a much-needed safety net.

Another vital aspect of preparing for independent living is encouraging your child to build a robust support network. This network should include family and friends who can offer emotional support, practical assistance, and professionals like therapists, counselors, or career advisors who can provide guidance tailored to your child's specific needs and challenges. This network will act as a pillar of strength and guidance, helping your child navigate the complexities of independent living more confidently and successfully.

Emphasize the importance of being flexible and adaptable. Plans may change, and that's okay. The ability to adjust and modify goals is a valuable life skill, especially for individuals with ADHD. Planning for independent living with your child is a process that requires patience, encouragement, and realistic goal-setting. It's about finding the right balance between providing support and allowing them to explore their independence. Working together, you can help your child with ADHD transition smoothly into a fulfilling and independent adult life.

As we conclude this chapter on fostering independence and responsibility in children with ADHD, it's clear that the journey toward independence is both challenging and rewarding. Parents can effectively guide their children toward a successful and independent adult life by exploring various educational paths, engaging in career exploration, and developing essential life skills. Setting realistic and achievable goals, providing necessary support and resources, and focusing on developing skills for further education, employment readiness, and financial independence are key steps in this process.

The importance of patience, understanding, and adaptability cannot be overstated. Each child with ADHD is unique, and their path to independence will be as individual as they are. The role of a parent in this journey is to provide a supportive and encouraging environment, helping their child realize their potential and confidently embrace their independence.

As we move on from discussing independence and responsibility, we find ourselves at the threshold of another critical aspect of development for children with ADHD: emotional regulation and well-being. The skills and confidence gained from fostering independence provide a solid foundation for tackling the complexities of emotional regulation.

In the next chapter, we will explore strategies and techniques to help children with ADHD understand and manage their emotions effectively, enhancing their overall well-being and ability to navigate life's challenges with resilience and grace. This next step is crucial, as emotional well-being is deeply intertwined with every child's growth and development aspect.

CHAPTER NINE

EMOTIONAL WELLBEING AND RESILIENCE

*I*magine a storm, unpredictable and powerful, with its strong gusts, torrential rains, and occasional spells of deceptive calm. This storm does not darken the sky but unfolds within the emotional landscape of a child with ADHD and their family. For parents and children grappling with ADHD, navigating these emotional ups and downs can often feel like steering a ship through such a turbulent sea. The gusts of anger, showers of frustration, and precious moments of calm are all parts of this intricate journey.

Living with ADHD is not just about managing attention and hyperactivity. It's also about understanding the whirlwind of emotions often accompanying this condition. These emotions can be intense, quick to surface, and challenging to control. For a child with ADHD, a minor setback can feel like a major catastrophe; a slight change in routine can trigger a storm of anxiety and resistance.

As parents, it's easy to feel overwhelmed and unequipped in the face of such emotional volatility. You may question your approach, wondering if you're too lenient, strict, involved, or distant. It's a balancing act that requires patience, understanding, and an ever-evolving set of strategies.

This chapter is dedicated to helping you understand and navigate these emotional complexities. We aim to provide you with practical strategies to enhance the emotional well-being and resilience of your child with ADHD. By delving into the nature of emotional triggers, the development of emotional intelligence, and the cultivation of resilience, we hope to empower you and your child to weather the storm more effectively. Navigating the emotional landscape of ADHD is not a journey that you or your child have to undertake alone. With the right understanding, tools, and support, you can turn this challenging journey into an opportunity for growth and connection. Let's embark on this journey together, learning to endure the storm and embrace and harness its power for positive change.

SECTION 1: IDENTIFYING TRIGGERS

Understanding your child's emotional experiences is the first step in navigating the complex world of ADHD. It's about peering beneath the often turbulent surface of their behaviors and recognizing the signs of emotional distress. Is their anger a mask for anxiety? Is frustration a sign of feeling misunderstood or overwhelmed? By identifying these emotional patterns and triggers, you can better anticipate and manage challenging situations, thus creating a more supportive and understanding environment for your child.

Identifying triggers is like learning a new language—the language of your child's emotions. This process involves keen observation, patience, and empathy. For children with ADHD, certain situations, environments, or demands can trigger intense emotional responses. These triggers can be external, like a noisy classroom, or internal, like feelings of inadequacy. Understanding these triggers helps in developing proactive strategies to reduce their impact.

UNDERSTANDING EMOTIONAL OUTBURSTS

Emotional outbursts in children with ADHD can often be sudden and intense. As a parent, it's crucial to understand what triggers these outbursts, as this knowledge is key to managing and eventually reducing their frequency and intensity. Common triggers include changes in routine, sensory overload, or feeling overwhelmed.

Children with ADHD often rely on routines to provide stability and predictability. Any deviation from their usual schedule can be disorienting, leading to frustration and emotional outbursts. Signs that your child is struggling with a change in routine might include increased agitation, resistance to new activities, or verbal outbursts when asked to transition from one activity to another.

Here are some tips for managing changes in routine:

Prepare in Advance: Prepare your child for upcoming changes whenever possible. Discuss what will happen and when, and reassure them about the process.

Visual Schedules: Visual schedules can illustrate the day's activities. This can help make abstract concepts more concrete for your child.

Gradual Transitions: Introduce changes slowly, allowing your child time to adjust to new routines.

Children with ADHD may be more sensitive to sensory stimuli such as noise, light, or touch. Sensory overload can occur when there's too much sensory information to process, leading to emotional outbursts as a way to escape the discomfort.

Signs of Sensory Overload

* Covering ears or eyes

* Irritability in crowded or loud environments

* Physical distress (e.g., headache, stomachache) in sensory-rich settings

Strategies to Reduce Sensory Overload

Sensory Breaks: Allow your child to take a break in a quiet, less stimulating environment.

Sensory Tools: Consider tools like noise-canceling headphones or fidget toys that can help manage sensory input.

Awareness of Environment: Be mindful of environments that might be overwhelming and plan visits during quieter times or provide coping strategies beforehand.

Children with ADHD can easily feel overwhelmed, especially when faced with tasks that seem large or complex. This can lead to emotional outbursts as a reaction to the stress and frustration of feeling unable to cope.

Signs to recognize an Overwhelmed Child:

* Procrastination or avoidance of certain tasks

* Expressing feelings of being unable to cope

* Breakdowns during homework or complex activities

TIPS FOR MANAGING FEELINGS OF OVERWHELM

Break Tasks into Smaller Steps: Help your child by breaking tasks into smaller, more manageable steps.

Encourage Verbalization of Feelings: Encourage your child to talk about their feelings of being overwhelmed. Understanding and verbalizing these emotions can be a powerful step in managing them.

Positive Reinforcement: Recognize and praise small accomplishments, boosting confidence and reducing overwhelming feelings. Understanding these triggers is just the first step. The next challenge lies in developing strategies to mitigate these triggers and teaching your child coping mechanisms to deal with them effectively. Remember, patience and consistency are key. As you learn more about your child's specific needs and triggers, you'll become better equipped to help them navigate their emotional world.

Strategies for Preventing Meltdowns

Once you have identified the triggers that lead to emotional outbursts in your child with ADHD, it's time to focus on strategies to prevent these meltdowns.

Here are some practical approaches:

Create a Structured Environment: Children with ADHD often thrive in structured environments. This doesn't mean rigid schedules but rather a predictable routine that provides security and reduces anxiety. Establish regular times for meals, homework, play, and bedtime. This predictability can significantly reduce stress. Use charts or visual aids to outline the day's activities. This can help your child understand what to expect next and prepare for transitions.

Use Visual Schedules: Visual schedules can be a game-changer for children with ADHD. Here are some ways they can be useful:

* Reducing Anxiety: Knowing what comes next reduces uncertainty and anxiety.

* Increasing Independence: They encourage children to take responsibility for their routines.

* Providing Clear Expectations: Visual schedules make abstract concepts concrete, especially for children with ADHD.

Teach Coping Strategies: Coping strategies are essential tools for your child to manage their emotions. Some effective strategies include:

* Deep Breathing: Teach your child deep breathing exercises. This can be a quick and effective way to calm down during moments of high stress or anxiety.

* Counting to Ten: Encourage your child to pause and count to ten when overwhelmed. This brief pause can help them regain control.

* Using a 'Calm Down' Space: Create a designated space in your home where your child can feel safe and relaxed. This could be a cozy corner with comforting items like soft pillows or favorite toys.

Encourage Physical Activity: Regular physical activity is crucial. It helps in managing energy levels and reduces stress. Encourage your child to play outside. Activities like running, jumping, or playing sports can be beneficial. Consider structured activities like martial arts or yoga, teaching discipline and focus.

Foster Open Communication and Positive Reinforcement: Encourage your child to express their feelings. When they can verbalize their feelings, it becomes easier to manage those emotions. Have daily check-ins to discuss feelings and concerns. Use emotion charts to help your child identify and articulate their feelings. Use positive reinforcement to encourage desired behaviors. This could be praise, a reward system, or simply acknowledging their efforts to manage their emotions.

Remember, every child is unique, and what works for one may not work for another. Be patient and try different strategies until you find the best for your child. Building these skills takes time, but you can help your child develop effective ways to prevent and manage meltdowns with consistent effort.

SUPPORTING EACH OTHER THROUGH CHALLENGES

Parenting a child with ADHD can often feel like a solitary journey, but it's important to remember that you're not alone. The support of others who understand your challenges can be incredibly uplifting and beneficial.

Here's how you can find and provide support to each other:

Joining Support Groups: Look for ADHD parent support groups in your community or online. These groups provide a platform to share experiences, tips, and resources. Engage in discussions, share your stories, and listen to others. Active participation can lead to deeper insights and more meaningful connections. Parents in these groups often have a wealth of knowledge about coping strategies, educational tips, and managing behavioral challenges. Their experiences can guide you in handling similar situations.

Connecting with Other Parents: Try to connect with parents in your child's school or neighborhood who are also raising children with ADHD. This network can be a source of immediate support and understanding. Exchange stories about what works and what doesn't. Sometimes, a strategy that worked for another family might be just what you need. These gatherings not only allow children to socialize and learn from each other but also give parents a chance to bond and discuss in a relaxed setting.

Providing Emotional Support: Sometimes, having someone to listen to you can make a big difference. Offer an empathetic ear to parents needing to express their feelings or discuss their challenges. Share your successes, no matter how small they may seem. This can provide hope and encouragement to others facing similar struggles. Celebrate the achievements of each other's children. Recognizing even minor progress can boost morale and foster a sense of community.

Leveraging Social Media and Online Forums: There are numerous online forums and social media groups dedicated to parents of children with ADHD. These can be great for getting advice or support at any time of the day. Use these platforms to share helpful articles, resources, and personal anecdotes. This information can be invaluable for parents seeking new ideas or solutions. Participate in virtual meetups, webinars, and workshops. These events can provide both learning opportunities and a sense of belonging.

Parenting a child with ADHD is a journey that you don't have to walk alone. You can build a supportive community around you and your child by joining hands with others who understand. This network provides practical help and emotional support and reminds you that your experiences are shared, valid, and understood.

SECTION 2: DEVELOPING EMOTIONAL INTELLIGENCE

Developing emotional intelligence in your child is another key aspect. This involves teaching them to recognize, name, and healthily express their feelings. It's about guiding them to understand their emotions, not as enemies, but as signals that must be interpreted and addressed. Role-playing, mindfulness, and meditation are some tools we'll explore to nurture this emotional awareness and regulation.

TEACHING HOW TO NAME AND EXPRESS FEELINGS

When it comes to helping your child with ADHD to navigate their emotional world, one of the most effective tools is teaching them to name and express their feelings. This process forms the bedrock of emotional intelligence, a vital skill for their overall development and well-being.

Begin with the basics. Introduce your child to simple, clear language to describe feelings. Words like *'happy,' 'sad,' 'angry,'* and *'scared'* are good starting points. Keep the language age-appropriate and straightforward. As mentioned, children with ADHD often respond well to visual stimuli. Utilize charts, emotion wheels, or flashcards with facial expressions representing different emotions. These aids can make the abstract concept of emotions more tangible and easier to understand.

Whenever your child experiences a strong emotion, help them label it. For instance, if they cry after a fall, say, *"It looks like you're feeling sad because you got hurt."* This consistent labeling helps them associate words with their feelings. Always validate their emotions, regardless of how trivial they might seem. Validation doesn't mean you agree with their feelings but acknowledge their right to feel that way. For example, *"I see you're upset because we can't go to the park today."*

Children learn a lot by imitation. Model healthy expression of emotions yourself. Show them it's okay to say, *"I am feeling stressed today,"* or *"I am really happy we spent the day together."* This modeling gives them a reference for expressing their own emotions.

Help your child understand what might trigger different emotions. Discuss situations from their daily life or stories and try to identify the emotions that these situations might evoke. This understanding can lead to better self-regulation. For older children, journaling can be a great way to express and understand emotions. For younger children, drawing can serve a similar purpose. Encourage them to draw or write about their feelings to process them.

Make it a routine to check in with your child about their feelings. You can do this at a certain time each day, like dinner or before bed. Ask them how they felt throughout the day and discuss why they might have felt that way.

If you find it challenging to help your child express their emotions, or if their emotional reactions seem extreme or unmanageable, don't hesitate to seek support from a child psychologist or therapist.

Teaching your child to name and express their feelings gives them a vital tool to manage their emotions effectively. This skill not only aids in their immediate emotional regulation but also lays the foundation for a healthy emotional life as they grow.

ROLE PLAYING EMOTIONAL RESPONSES

Role-playing is a dynamic and effective tool for helping children with ADHD develop better emotional responses. It's a method that allows children to practice dealing with various emotional scenarios in a safe, controlled, and, importantly, non-judgmental setting. This approach can significantly aid in enhancing their emotional intelligence and response strategies.

Here are key components and strategies for implementing role-playing in your daily interactions:

Creating Scenarios: Create scenarios your child will likely encounter. These can range from dealing with disappointment and frustration to expressing joy and excitement appropriately. The scenarios should be relatable and tailored to your child's experiences. For example, how to react when they don't win a game or express themselves when they need help with schoolwork.

Role Reversal: A powerful aspect of role-playing involves reversing roles. Allow your child to play the role of the parent, teacher, or friend. This helps them see situations from another perspective, fostering empathy and understanding. It also gives you insight into how your child perceives the reactions of others.

Guided Practice: Guide your child through appropriate emotional responses during role-playing. If they struggle to find the right words or actions, offer suggestions and model behavior for them. This guided practice helps in embedding constructive emotional responses.

Feedback and Discussion: After each role-playing session, discuss what went well and what could be improved. Offer positive reinforcement for efforts and progress, not just for *'correct'* responses. Encourage your child to express their feelings during the role-play and what they think they could do differently in real situations.

Emphasizing Non-Verbal Cues: Teach your child to understand and respond to non-verbal cues like facial expressions and body language. Role-playing provides a great opportunity to practice interpreting these cues in a controlled setting.

Incorporating Real-life Situations: Gradually incorporate scenarios that mirror real-life situations your child recently experienced. Discuss how they handled the situation and how they might handle it differently. This reflection can lead to tangible improvements in real-life interactions.

Using Props and Visual Aids: To make the role-play more engaging and realistic, use props and visual aids. These can be simple items from around the house or pictures and charts that help illustrate emotional states.

Regular Practice: Incorporate role-playing regularly into your routine. Consistent practice helps children with ADHD apply these skills automatically in real life, improving their emotional responses.

Building a Supportive Environment: Creating a supportive and understanding environment during these exercises is essential. Make it clear that it's a safe space to express emotions and that making mistakes is part of the learning process.

Role-playing is not just about teaching your child what to do in specific situations; it's about giving them the tools to understand and manage their emotions effectively. They can learn to navigate emotions through regular practice, improving interactions and emotional well-being.

THE ROLE OF MINDFULNESS AND MEDITATION

Mindfulness and meditation, often perceived as tranquil practices, hold significant promise for parents and children dealing with ADHD. These practices are not just about finding a quiet moment in a busy day; they are powerful tools for cultivating a sense of calm, improving focus, and enhancing emotional regulation.

Mindfulness is a state of active, open attention to the present moment. It involves observing thoughts, feelings, and sensations without judgment. On the other hand, meditation is a practice where an individual uses a technique – such as focusing their mind on a particular object, thought, or activity – to achieve a mentally clear and emotionally calm state.

Mindfulness practices teach children to pay attention in a particular way, on purpose, in the present moment. This skill is especially beneficial for children with ADHD, who often struggle with maintaining focus. Regular mindfulness and meditation can help children become more aware of their emotions, understand them better, and respond to them more thoughtfully rather than reacting impulsively.

Mindfulness practices teach children to pay attention in a particular way, on purpose, in the present moment. This skill is especially beneficial for children with ADHD, who often struggle with maintaining focus. Regular mindfulness and meditation can help children become more aware of their emotions, understand them better, and respond to them more thoughtfully rather than reacting impulsively.

Here's how to Integrate Mindfulness and Meditation into Daily Life:

Start with Short Sessions: Start with just a few minutes daily and gradually increase the duration. Even brief periods of mindfulness can be beneficial.

Use Guided Practices: Guided meditations can be more engaging for beginners, especially children. Many apps and online resources are available with guided sessions specifically designed for children.

Incorporate Mindful Moments: Encourage your child to have mindful moments throughout the day. This could be as simple as taking deep breaths before starting a task or noticing the sensations while eating.

Practice Together: Engage in mindfulness or meditation practices as a family. This not only provides support but also establishes a routine.

Be Consistent: Like any other skill, mindfulness and meditation require consistent practice. Encourage your child to stick with it, even if it's just for a few minutes each day.

Make it Fun: For younger children, turn mindfulness into a game. Use imaginative scenarios or fun activities like mindful listening to sounds in the environment or mindful coloring.

Introducing mindfulness and meditation into your child's life can be a transformative experience. These practices offer a way to navigate the tumultuous waters of ADHD with more grace and less stress. Remember, the goal is not to empty the mind of thoughts but to learn how to observe them without getting swept away. By fostering these skills, you are equipping your child with a valuable tool for life that transcends beyond managing ADHD symptoms to enhancing overall well-being.

SECTION 3: BUILDING RESILIENCE

The ability to bounce back from setbacks is crucial for any child, but it's especially vital for those with ADHD. We'll discuss strategies to help your child develop a growth mindset, see challenges as opportunities for learning, and find joy and self-esteem in their hobbies and passions.

STRATEGIES FOR BOUNCING BACK FROM SETBACKS

Setbacks, though challenging, are an integral part of growth, especially for children with ADHD. These moments, when approached correctly, can become powerful learning opportunities.

The following are some strategies to help your child bounce back from setbacks, fostering resilience and a positive mindset:

Embrace a Growth Mindset: Begin by teaching your child that setbacks are not failures but opportunities to learn and grow. Emphasize that skills and abilities can be developed through effort and perseverance. When encountering a setback, encourage them to ask, *"What can I learn from this?"* rather than dwelling on the disappointment.

Problem-Solving Together: When a setback occurs, sit down with your child and engage in a problem-solving session. Break down the problem into smaller, manageable parts. Ask questions like, *"What was the challenge?"*, *"What strategies did we try?"* and *"What could we do differently next time?"* This approach helps find solutions and teaches your child a structured approach to difficulties.

Celebrate Efforts, Not Just Outcomes: Praise your child for their effort, not just the outcome. Regardless of the result, celebrating the hard work they put into a task reinforces the value of trying and learning from the experience. This builds their confidence and encourages them to keep trying in the face of challenges.

Teach Resilience Through Role Models: Share stories of real or fictional people who have overcome obstacles. Discussing how these individuals faced challenges and bounced back can be incredibly motivating. It can also provide practical examples of resilience in action.

Reflective Conversations: Engage in a reflective conversation with your child after a setback. Discuss what happened, how they felt, and what thoughts went through their mind. This reflection can provide insights into their emotional response and thought processes, helping them develop greater self-awareness and coping strategies.

Encourage a Routine of Reflection: Establish a routine where your child reflects on their day or week. Have them identify what went well and what was challenging. This regular practice of reflection helps children recognize patterns in their experiences and learn from them.

Foster Independence: While supporting your child is important, remember that encouraging independence is equally crucial. Allow them to attempt to solve problems on their own before stepping in. This independence builds confidence and resilience as they learn they can handle challenges.

Maintain a Positive Environment: Create an environment where it's safe to make mistakes. A supportive and non-judgmental atmosphere at home encourages children to take risks, try new things, and learn from their experiences without fear of criticism.

These strategies are not just tools for handling setbacks; they are lessons in life skills that your child with ADHD will carry into adulthood. By teaching them to see challenges as opportunities, you're equipping them with the resilience and mindset to navigate the complexities of life with confidence and optimism.

THE POWER OF A GROWTH MINDSET

One of the most empowering gifts you can give your child, especially one with ADHD, is the perspective of a growth mindset. This concept, popularized by psychologist Carol Dweck, is based on the belief that dedication and hard work can develop abilities and intelligence. For children with ADHD, who often face unique learning challenges and frequent setbacks, embracing a growth mindset can be transformative.

Let's distinguish it from a fixed mindset before we delve into fostering a growth mindset. A fixed mindset assumes that our character, intelligence, and creative abilities are static, given that we can't change meaningfully. In contrast, a growth mindset thrives on challenge and sees failure not as evidence of unintelligence but as a springboard for growth and stretching our existing abilities.

Here are some Strategies to Cultivate a Growth Mindset:

Praise the Process, Not Just the Outcome: Focus on your child's effort into a task, rather than just praising them for their innate abilities. Statements like *"I'm proud of how hard you worked on this"* or *"Your dedication shows in your work"* highlight the value of perseverance and effort.

Encourage Perseverance: Children with ADHD may get frustrated and give up easily. Encourage them to persist with challenging tasks, offering support and guidance. This might involve breaking down tasks into smaller, more manageable steps or setting incremental goals.

Model a Growth Mindset: Children learn by example. Demonstrate your own growth mindset by discussing your challenges and how you overcome them. Share your learning experiences and how you persist through difficulties.

Teach the Brain's Ability to Grow: Explain to your child that their brain is like a muscle that gets stronger and smarter the more it's used. Discuss neuroplasticity – the brain's ability to change and adapt due to experience – to reinforce this concept.

Use Growth-Minded Language: Our language can shape our thinking. Use phrases that promote a growth mindset, like *"You can learn to do this"* or *"This may take some time and effort,"* instead of fixed mindset phrases like *"You're just not good at this."*

Set Learning Goals: Learning goals, rather than performance goals, can help shift the focus from proving an ability to improving it. These goals involve acquiring new skills or knowledge rather than achieving a specific grade or score.

Celebrate Improvements: Recognize and celebrate improvements, no matter how small. This reinforces the idea that progress is a significant achievement.

Adopting a growth mindset can be particularly beneficial for children with ADHD. It helps them see challenges as opportunities for development, makes them resilient in the face of adversity, and encourages a lifelong love of learning. As a parent, your support and guidance in developing this mindset can profoundly impact your child's perception of themselves and their abilities, paving the way for success and fulfillment in many areas of their lives.

ENCOURAGING HOBBIES AND PASSIONS

Engaging in hobbies and passions is not just a pastime; for children with ADHD, it can be a vital therapeutic activity. Immersing themselves in a hobby they love provides a constructive outlet for their boundless energy and creativity. This engagement can be fulfilling and rewarding, offering them a sense of achievement and joy they might not find in more structured or academic settings.

Hobbies and passions, ranging from painting and music to sports and technology, allow children to explore and express themselves in a setting free from the pressures of performance or judgment. It's a space where they can set their own pace, explore their interests, and develop a deep sense of personal satisfaction and accomplishment. The success experienced in these areas can be a significant confidence booster, helping them to feel more competent and capable.

Moreover, pursuing hobbies has the added benefit of developing new skills and talents. For a child with ADHD, this skill development happens in a context where they are motivated and engaged, which can make learning more effective and enjoyable. It's also an opportunity for parents to bond with their children, sharing their interests and celebrating their achievements.

Incorporating hobbies and passions into the daily routine of a child with ADHD can also serve as a calming and stabilizing factor. These activities can provide a natural and enjoyable structure for the child. It's a chance for them to take control and make choices about how they spend their time, giving them a sense of autonomy and independence.

Parents must encourage and support their children's hobbies and passions, even if they change frequently. This exploration is a natural part of any child's learning and growth process, especially for those with ADHD. Encouraging them to follow their interests nurtures their emotional well-being and helps them discover their strengths and potential. In doing so, we provide them with a valuable tool for coping with the challenges of ADHD, enabling them to find joy, purpose, and success in their own unique way.

As we conclude this chapter on enhancing emotional well-being and resilience, it's important to recognize our progress. We've explored ways to identify emotional triggers, develop emotional intelligence, and build resilience in our children with ADHD. These tools are invaluable in helping them navigate their emotional world. However, our journey doesn't end here.

In the next and final chapter, we will examine the intricacies of the healthcare system, a crucial aspect of supporting our child's overall development and well-being. Navigating this system can be daunting, but understanding its various components and how to access them effectively is essential. We will explore how to partner with healthcare professionals, understand different treatment options, and advocate for your child's unique needs. This knowledge will empower you to make informed decisions, ensuring your child receives the comprehensive support they deserve.

Let's move forward together, equipped with a strengthened emotional toolkit and a readiness to engage with the healthcare landscape to provide the best possible care for our children.

CHAPTER TEN

NAVIGATING HEALTHCARE AND SUPPORT SYSTEMS

*W*hen it comes to parenting a child with ADHD, the role you play can make a significant difference in their life. Are you actively advocating for their needs, or are you on the sidelines, unsure how to navigate the complex world of healthcare and support systems? This is a question many parents face, often overwhelmed by the array of decisions and options available.

Parenting is a journey filled with challenges and triumphs, and when your child has ADHD, this journey takes on additional layers of complexity. From understanding the nuances of the condition to finding the right healthcare professionals, from exploring therapy options to accessing community support, the path is intricate and often daunting.

This chapter empowers you, the parent, to become a proactive and informed advocate for your child. The reality of ADHD is that it doesn't just affect the child; it impacts the entire family and your approach to parenting. Equipping yourself with knowledge and strategies allows you to transition from feeling like a bystander to being a confident advocate.

We will explore how to partner effectively with healthcare professionals, understanding the significance of choosing providers who are knowledgeable about ADHD. The journey includes educating yourself and your loved ones and creating a supportive network for your child. We'll delve into the various aspects of medication and therapy, offering a balanced view of available options. Furthermore, this chapter will guide you through the wealth of community resources, from local support groups to educational workshops, and help you navigate the financial and legal aspects of ADHD care.

Embarking on this path is about more than just managing a condition; it's about enriching your child's life despite the challenges of ADHD. It's about advocating for their best interests and ensuring they have the tools and support they need to thrive. As you read through this chapter, remember that your role is pivotal. You have the power to make a significant impact on your child's journey with ADHD.

SECTION 1: CHOOSING THE RIGHT PROVIDERS

Navigating the healthcare landscape for a child with ADHD can be a daunting task. It is critical to find providers who are not only knowledgeable about ADHD but also align with your child's unique needs. This section is designed to guide you through choosing the right healthcare professionals. We will explore the importance of finding ADHD-knowledgeable providers, how to educate your loved ones about ADHD, and the benefits of a multidisciplinary team approach. By the end of this section, you will have a clearer understanding of creating a supportive and effective healthcare team for your child.

FINDING ADHD-KNOWLEDGEABLE PROFESSIONALS

When your child is diagnosed with Attention Deficit Hyperactivity Disorder (ADHD), the journey ahead can seem daunting. One of the first and most important steps is finding the right healthcare professionals specializing in ADHD. This decision can significantly affect how effectively your child's condition is managed and treated.

Professionals with a specialization in ADHD have a deep understanding of the condition, which goes beyond the basic knowledge that general practitioners may have. ADHD is a complex neurodevelopmental disorder that affects each child uniquely. Specialists in this field are equipped to recognize the nuances of ADHD, including how it can present differently in children and evolve over time.

These professionals are familiar with the range of symptoms and behaviors associated with ADHD, such as inattention, hyperactivity, and impulsivity, and how these can impact different aspects of life, including school performance, social interactions, and family dynamics. Their comprehensive understanding allows them to diagnose ADHD accurately, an essential step since ADHD can often be mistaken for other behavioral or emotional issues.

ADHD research and treatment strategies are constantly evolving. Professionals dedicated to this field are typically abreast of the latest developments, be it new medications, behavioral therapies, or holistic approaches. This up-to-date knowledge ensures that your child can access the most current and effective treatment options.

Such professionals can also provide guidance on managing ADHD symptoms in various settings, like at home or school, and suggest modifications or accommodations that can help your child succeed. They can work closely with your child's school to implement individualized education plans (IEPs) or 504 plans designed to provide support and accommodations in the educational environment.

Every child with ADHD is unique, and what works for one child may not work for another. ADHD-knowledgeable professionals can tailor their advice and treatment plans to fit your child's needs. They consider various factors like the child's age, the severity of symptoms, coexisting conditions, and family dynamics.

These experts also understand the importance of a holistic approach to treatment, which might include a combination of medication, behavioral therapy, lifestyle changes, and support for emotional and social challenges. They are skilled in working collaboratively with families, understanding their concerns, and providing support and guidance through the challenges of raising a child with ADHD.

In summary, seeking healthcare professionals who specialize in ADHD is a critical step in ensuring your child receives the best possible care. These experts' deep understanding of ADHD, knowledge of the latest treatment options, and ability to provide tailored support can significantly impact your child's quality of life and overall development. As a parent, partnering with the right healthcare professional is a vital component in the journey of supporting and advocating for your child with ADHD.

EDUCATING LOVED ONES ABOUT ADHD

When your child has ADHD, the understanding and support of your family and friends can make a significant difference in their life and development. However, ADHD is often misunderstood, leading to misconceptions and ineffective responses from those close to the child. Here, we discuss how to effectively communicate about ADHD with your loved ones to foster a supportive and informed environment.

Start with the basics and explain that Attention Deficit Hyperactivity Disorder (ADHD) is a neurodevelopmental disorder, not a result of poor parenting or lack of discipline. Symptoms like inattention, hyperactivity, and impulsivity characterize it. Emphasize that ADHD affects each child differently, and symptoms can vary in intensity.

Use specific examples from your child's life to illustrate ADHD in daily scenarios. This could include difficulty concentrating on tasks, difficulty sitting still, or acting impulsively. Personal stories make ADHD more relatable and help others understand your child's unique experiences.

Many myths about ADHD can lead to misunderstandings. Take time to debunk these myths. For example, ADHD is not just about being hyperactive; it also involves challenges with concentration and self-regulation. Also, clarify that ADHD is not just a childhood condition; many continue to experience symptoms into adulthood.

Explain how ADHD affects academic performance, social interactions, and self-esteem. Discuss your child's frustrations and challenges, such as difficulties making friends or feeling overwhelmed by schoolwork. This helps loved ones understand the broader impact of ADHD.

Encourage your family and friends to approach your child with empathy and patience. Explain that children with ADHD often need extra time to process information and may require different approaches to learning and communication. Offer resources for those who want to learn more about ADHD. This can include books, websites, and articles that offer deeper insights into the condition. Consider suggesting online forums or support groups where they can hear from others affected by ADHD.

Discuss what has been effective in supporting your child. This might include structured routines, clear and consistent rules, or specific types of positive reinforcement. Encourage loved ones to use these strategies to create a consistent support system for your child.

Finally, invite your family and friends to ask questions and express their thoughts and concerns. An open dialogue clears misunderstandings and helps everyone be on the same page in supporting your child. By educating your loved ones about ADHD, you're advocating for your child and building a supportive network that can positively impact your child's growth and self-esteem.

THE MULTI-DISCIPLINARY TEAM APPROACH

When managing ADHD, a multidisciplinary team approach can be highly effective. This method involves assembling a group of professionals from various fields who collaborate to address the diverse needs of a child with ADHD. Each team member brings unique expertise and insights, contributing to a more comprehensive treatment plan. Below, we'll explore how to build and utilize this team for the benefit of your child.

Pediatricians or Child Psychiatrists: These medical professionals are often the first point of contact. They can diagnose ADHD, prescribe and manage medications, and monitor the child's overall health. They provide a medical perspective on ADHD and its impact on the child's physical well-being.

Psychologists or Psychiatrists: Psychologists assess behavioral and emotional issues and provide therapy. Psychiatrists, while also capable of providing treatment, can prescribe medications. They play a crucial role in addressing the psychological aspects of ADHD, such as anxiety or depression, that often accompany the disorder.

Special Education Teachers or School Counselors: These educators understand the educational implications of ADHD. They can develop and implement Individualized Education Plans (IEPs) or 504 Plans to provide academic accommodations and support in the school environment.

Behavioral Therapists: These therapists specialize in teaching children with ADHD strategies to manage their symptoms. Cognitive Behavioral Therapy (CBT) or behavior modification strategies are common. They work closely with the child to develop practical skills for everyday challenges.

Occupational Therapists: If your child has sensory processing issues or struggles with fine motor skills, an occupational therapist can be invaluable. They help develop these skills and make daily life's physical aspects more manageable for a child with ADHD.

Speech-Language Pathologists: If there are concerns about your child's communication skills, a speech-language pathologist can assess and assist in this area. They address issues related to language, speech, and communication.

When coordinating your team, the following should be prioritized:

Open Communication: Ensure regular and open communication among team members. Sharing insights and progress across different areas provides a more complete picture of your child's needs and development.

Regular Meetings: Organize periodic meetings with the team, in-person or virtually, to discuss plans, set goals, and review progress. This helps keep everyone on the same page and allows for adjustments in strategies as needed.

Your Role as the Parent: As a parent, you are an integral part of this team. Share your observations, concerns, and insights about your child. Your input is valuable in shaping the approach the team takes.

Involving Your Child: Depending on their age and understanding, involve your child in discussions and decisions. This fosters a sense of responsibility and empowerment in them.

To utilize the team effectively, work toward clear, achievable goals for your child. These should cover various aspects such as academic achievement, behavior management, social skills, and emotional well-being. Encourage team members to integrate their approaches. For example, a therapist's recommendations can be supported at school and at home. Monitor and regularly monitor your child's progress, evaluate the effectiveness of the implemented strategies, and be open to making changes as necessary.

Remember that ADHD affects the entire family. Some team members, like psychologists, can provide support and guidance for siblings and parents, helping the family unit navigate the challenges of ADHD together. By effectively building and coordinating a multidisciplinary team, you can create a robust support system tailored to your child's unique needs, ensuring they have the best possible foundation for managing ADHD and thriving in all areas of their life.

SECTION 2: MEDICATION AND THERAPY

Medication and therapy form the cornerstone of ADHD management. However, understanding and navigating these options can often be overwhelming. This section provides an overview of ADHD medications, including how to manage them effectively, and delves into the various forms of behavioral therapy and their benefits. We will also discuss alternative therapies and their role in a comprehensive treatment plan. Our goal is to provide a balanced and comprehensive understanding of these treatment options, enabling you to make informed decisions that best suit your child's needs.

OVERVIEW OF ADHD MEDICATIONS AND THEIR MANAGEMENT

Medication can be a crucial component of ADHD treatment. It's important to understand that while medication doesn't cure ADHD, it can significantly help manage its symptoms. This section will provide an overview of common ADHD medications, their potential side effects, and tips for managing these medications effectively.

Stimulants are the most commonly prescribed medications for

ADHD. They increase and balance levels of neurotransmitters in the brain. Non-stimulants can be used when stimulants are ineffective or cause severe side effects. They take longer to start working than stimulants but can have a smoother effect.

While medications can be effective, they can also come with side effects. It is important to monitor and communicate with your healthcare provider about these side effects.

Common side effects of stimulants include:

 * Decreased appetite

 * Insomnia

 * Increased heart rate

 * Headaches

 * Mood swings

Non-stimulants may cause:

 * Fatigue

 * Nausea

 * Dizziness

 * Mood changes

Tips for Managing Medications Effectively

Consistent Communication with Your Healthcare Provider: Regular check-ins with your doctor are crucial. They can adjust dosages, change medications, and help manage side effects.

Detailed Monitoring: Monitor any side effects and how the medication affects your child's behavior and mood. This information is invaluable for your healthcare provider.

Medication Timing: Be attentive to the timing of medication. Some should be taken in the morning to avoid insomnia, while others might need to be taken at specific times during the day.

Understanding Medication Breaks: Some parents and healthcare providers consider "drug holidays" or breaks from ADHD medication. Discuss this option with your doctor to determine if it's appropriate for your child.

Education About Medication: Educate yourself and your child about the medication. Understanding why and how it helps can make managing it easier.

Be Aware of Potential Misuse: Particularly with stimulants, there's a risk of misuse. Store medication safely and discuss the importance of taking it as prescribed.

Lifestyle Integration: Combine medication with behavioral therapy, a healthy diet, exercise, and sufficient sleep for the best results.

Medicating is a significant decision and should be made with thorough consultation with your healthcare provider. Remember, medication is just one part of a comprehensive treatment plan for ADHD. With careful management and a holistic approach, medication can be an effective tool in helping your child manage their ADHD symptoms.

BEHAVIORAL THERAPY AND ITS BENEFITS

Behavioral therapy is a vital part of the treatment plan for children with Attention Deficit Hyperactivity Disorder (ADHD). This therapy focuses on changing specific behaviors by reinforcing desired behaviors and reducing unwanted ones. It's particularly effective for children with ADHD because it addresses the challenges they face in behavior management, impulse control, and social interaction.

Behavioral therapy for ADHD involves structured interventions designed to modify specific aspects of a child's behavior. This therapy can occur in various settings, including at home, in school, or in a clinical environment. It often involves close collaboration between therapists, parents, teachers, and the child.

Here are Some Different Types of Behavioral Therapies

Behavior Modification: Involves using a rewards system to encourage positive behavior and consequences to discourage negative behavior. This method helps children understand the direct outcomes of their actions.

Cognitive-Behavioral Therapy (CBT): CBT helps children identify negative thought patterns and replace them with more positive, constructive thinking. This therapy is effective in managing the emotional challenges associated with ADHD.

Social Skills Training: This therapy focuses on improving social interactions. It teaches children how to read social cues, understand others' emotions, and respond appropriately in social settings.

Parent Training: Therapists work with parents to teach them strategies for managing their child's behavior. This includes learning how to give effective instructions, setting boundaries, and using rewards and consequences.

School-Based Interventions: These interventions involve teachers and school counselors. Strategies include behavior plans, adjustments in teaching methods, and accommodations to help the child succeed academically.

Here are Some Benefits of Behavioral Therapy:

* Behavioral therapy helps children learn techniques to increase their attention span and control impulsive behaviors.

* As children learn to read and respond to social cues, they find it easier to make friends and interact with peers and adults.

* Children learn to manage disruptive behaviors, such as outbursts and aggression, by understanding the consequences of their actions.

* Successfully managing their symptoms can boost children's confidence and self-esteem.

* When parents are involved in therapy, it improves communication and understanding within the family, leading to stronger relationships.

* The skills learned in behavioral therapy are not just for childhood; they provide a foundation for managing ADHD symptoms throughout life.

Behavioral therapy is a powerful tool in managing ADHD. It equips children with the skills to navigate their symptoms and challenges, improving their behavior, social interactions, and overall well-being. Your involvement and support in this process are crucial as a parent, providing a consistent and nurturing environment for your child to thrive.

ALTERNATIVE THERAPIES AND THEIR PLACE IN TREATMENT

While traditional treatments such as medication and behavioral therapy are often at the forefront of ADHD management, alternative therapies can also play a significant role in supporting your child. Integrating these complementary approaches can enhance overall well-being and symptom management. This section explores several alternative therapies, including dietary modifications, exercise, and mindfulness practices, and how they can bolster traditional ADHD treatments.

Research suggests that specific dietary changes can help manage ADHD symptoms. While no specific "ADHD diet" works for everyone, some general guidelines may be beneficial:

Reducing Sugar and Processed Foods: High sugar intake

and processed foods can exacerbate hyperactivity and concentration issues in some children.

Omega-3 Fatty Acids: Omega-3s, found in fish, flaxseeds, and walnuts, are known for their brain health benefits and may improve attention spans.

Balanced Meals: A diet balanced in proteins, carbohydrates, and healthy fats can help maintain steady energy levels and mood throughout the day.

Before making significant dietary changes, consulting with a nutritionist or healthcare provider is recommended. They can help tailor a nutrition plan that suits your child's needs and ensures they receive all necessary nutrients.

Physical activity is not just beneficial for physical health; it also profoundly impacts mental well-being. For children with ADHD, regular exercise can lead to improvements in:

* Concentration and attention

* Mood regulation

* Reduction in anxiety and depression symptoms

* Better sleep patterns

Finding activities your child enjoys is key to maintaining a consistent exercise routine. This can include team sports, martial arts, dance, or simply playing outdoors. The goal is to make physical activity a fun and regular part of their life.

Mindfulness exercises has been gaining a lot of attention as an effective tool for managing ADHD symptoms. It involves being present in the moment. Practices like meditation, yoga, and deep breathing can help children with ADHD to:

* Improve focus and attention

* Reduce impulsivity

* Manage stress and anxiety

* Enhance self-awareness

Start with short, guided mindfulness exercises suited for children. Many resources are available, including apps, online videos, and books designed to engage children in mindfulness practices.

While these alternative therapies can be beneficial, they are usually most effective when used in conjunction with traditional ADHD treatments. Maintaining open communication with your child's healthcare team and integrating these alternative methods as part of a broader treatment plan is important. Alternative therapies offer a range of benefits that can complement traditional ADHD treatments. Incorporating dietary changes, exercise, and mindfulness into your child's routine can provide them with additional tools to manage their symptoms and improve their overall quality of life. Remember, each child is unique, so finding the right combination of treatments that work best for your child's needs is essential.

SECTION 3: ASSESSING COMMUNITY RESOURCES

Beyond the realms of medication and therapy, there exists a wealth of community resources that can be invaluable in supporting your child with ADHD. This section will explore how to find and utilize these resources, including local and online support groups, educational resources and workshops, and avenues for financial assistance and legal rights. Understanding and accessing these resources can provide additional layers of support, not just for your child but for your entire family. This section aims to equip you with the knowledge to tap into these resources, enhancing your ability to support and advocate for your child effectively.

LOCAL AND ONLINE SUPPORT GROUPS

Support groups play a pivotal role in the journey of parenting a child with ADHD. They provide information, emotional support, understanding, and a sense of belonging. In these groups, you'll find parents who share similar challenges and triumphs, creating a community that understands your journey intimately. Local support groups can be found through various channels:

Schools and Educational Institutions: Often, schools have resources or can direct you to local groups that support children with ADHD and their families.

Hospitals and Clinics: Pediatricians or ADHD specialists may have information about support groups in your area.

Community Centers: Local community centers, libraries, and religious institutions often host or have information about support groups.

ADHD Organizations: National and regional ADHD organizations often have listings of local support groups on their websites.

When attending local support groups, expect a mix of structured activities like discussions, guest speakers, and informal gatherings.

These meetings offer a chance to connect personally with other parents, exchange stories, and learn from each other's experiences.

Online support groups offer flexibility and a wider community, accessible from the comfort of your home.

Here's how to find them:

Social Media Platforms: Facebook, Reddit, and Instagram have numerous ADHD support groups. These can range from general ADHD support to more specific focuses, like parenting children with ADHD.

Forums and Websites: Websites dedicated to ADHD often host forums where you can ask questions, share experiences, and receive support.

Online Meetups: Websites can have virtual groups, offering a more structured environment for support and discussion.

Blogs and Online Communities: Blogs focused on ADHD often have associated communities where readers can interact and support each other.

Both local and online support groups can be invaluable resources for parents of children with ADHD. They offer a platform for learning, sharing, and finding emotional solace in a community that understands your journey. By engaging with these groups, you can discover new strategies, insights, and the reassurance that you are not alone in this journey.

EDUCATIONAL RESOURCES AND WORKSHOPS

Parenting a child with ADHD is a journey that often requires continuous learning and adaptation. Educational resources and workshops are invaluable tools in this process, offering insights, strategies, and a deeper understanding of effectively managing ADHD. Here, we explore how to access and utilize these resources, including online courses, books, and seminars.

Online courses are a flexible and convenient way to learn about ADHD. They allow you to study at your own pace, on your own schedule, and often provide a wide range of topics. Websites like Coursera, Udemy, and Khan Academy offer courses designed by experts in the field. These courses cover various aspects of ADHD, including its neurobiological basis, behavioral strategies, and practical parenting tips.

A wealth of books on ADHD are available, written by experts, educators, and even parents with firsthand experience. These books can provide comprehensive information, from understanding the science behind ADHD to practical day-to-day management strategies. Make sure to consider the books listed in our sources list. Local libraries, bookstores, and online retailers like Amazon are good places to find these books. Also, consider audiobooks or eBooks if they fit your lifestyle better.

Attending seminars and workshops can be highly beneficial. These events often bring together ADHD experts, educators, and other parents, providing a platform for learning and discussion. They can offer the latest research findings, practical strategies, and the opportunity to ask questions directly to experts. Some organizations offer workshops specifically designed for children with ADHD. These workshops focus on helping children understand their condition, learn coping strategies, and build social skills. They can be an excellent way for your child to meet others facing similar challenges.

Finally, consider seeking out schools or educational programs that have a strong focus on supporting children with ADHD. These environments can be more conducive to your child's learning and development needs.

The wealth of educational resources and workshops available for parents of children with ADHD is vast and varied. By taking advantage of these resources, you can better understand ADHD and learn effective strategies to support your child's growth and success. Remember, the journey of parenting a child with ADHD is one of continual learning and adaptation, and these resources can be your guide and support along the way.

FINANCIAL ASSISTANCE AND LEGAL RIGHTS

Navigating the financial and legal aspects of ADHD care can be overwhelming. However, understanding these areas is crucial to ensure your child receives the best possible support and accommodations. This section will guide you through navigating insurance, seeking financial assistance, and understanding your child's legal rights in the educational system.

Understanding Your Coverage: Review your health insurance policy thoroughly. Understand what treatments, therapies, and medications are covered under your plan. Look for specific clauses related to mental health and behavioral disorders.

Pre-Authorizations and Referrals: Some insurance plans require pre-authorization for certain treatments or referrals from a primary care physician. Be aware of these requirements to avoid unexpected costs.

Appealing Denials: You can appeal if your insurance denies coverage for a particular treatment or medication. Gather medical evidence and letters from healthcare providers to support your appeal.

Seeking financial assistance for ADHD-related expenses can be a crucial step for many families. A primary avenue to explore is government-funded programs like Medicaid or the Children's Health Insurance Program (CHIP). These programs can provide additional coverage, especially useful if your current insurance does not fully cover the needs of your child's ADHD treatment.

Another resource to consider is pharmaceutical assistance programs offered by many drug companies. These programs are designed to help reduce the cost of medications, which can be a significant relief for families managing the expenses of ADHD medications. It's worth researching and applying to these programs, as they can make a substantial difference in the affordability of necessary treatments.

Additionally, there are grants and scholarships specifically aimed at families with children who have ADHD. Organizations like CHADD (Children and Adults with Attention-Deficit/ Hyperactivity Disorder) are valuable resources for finding such financial aid. They often provide links and information about available grants and scholarships, which can help offset the costs associated with managing ADHD.

Lastly, some therapists and clinics offer sliding scale fees for therapy and consultations. These fees are adjusted based on a family's income, making treatment more accessible and affordable. It's important not to hesitate to inquire about this option, as many healthcare providers are willing to work with families to ensure that necessary treatments are not financially prohibitive. This approach ensures that financial constraints do not prevent your child from receiving the best possible care and support.

Legal Rights in the Educational System:

Individuals with Disabilities Education Act (IDEA): Under IDEA, children with disabilities, including ADHD, are entitled to Free Appropriate Public Education (FAPE). This may include special education services, individualized education programs (IEP), and accommodations.

504 Plans: Section 504 of the Rehabilitation Act of 1973 allows students with disabilities to have accommodations in the regular classroom setting. For children with ADHD, this could include extended time on tests, reduced homework or classwork, and preferential seating.

Advocating for Your Child: Become an advocate for your child in their school. Work with teachers, school counselors, and administrators to meet your child's needs. It's essential to keep detailed records of meetings and communications.

Seeking Legal Advice: If you face challenges obtaining the necessary accommodations or services for your child, consider consulting with an attorney specializing in education law.

Remember, understanding and utilizing these financial and legal resources can alleviate some burdens of managing ADHD. It empowers you to advocate effectively for your child, ensuring they receive the necessary support to succeed academically and in their personal growth.

As we conclude this chapter on navigating healthcare and support systems for your child with ADHD, it's essential to reflect on how each element we've discussed fits into a more extensive, holistic approach to parenting. ADHD, with its unique challenges and nuances, requires a comprehensive strategy that encompasses medical, psychological, educational, and familial aspects. This holistic approach is about creating a supportive ecosystem that caters to your child's specific needs, enabling them to thrive both at home and in the wider world.

The journey starts with choosing the right healthcare professionals who understand ADHD and can offer tailored care. Medications, if prescribed, should be managed carefully, balancing efficacy with any potential side effects. Alongside medical treatment, behavioral therapy is crucial in developing coping mechanisms and social skills. Remember, this combination of medical and therapeutic care forms the backbone of your child's support system, addressing both the symptoms and the underlying challenges of ADHD.

Your role in educating teachers and school administrators about your child's needs is vital. Advocating for appropriate accommodations ensures that your child has a fair and supportive learning environment. Furthermore, engaging with community resources, such as support groups and workshops, can offer additional layers of support for your child and you as a parent. These resources provide a platform for shared experiences, advice, and emotional support, enriching your understanding and approach to ADHD parenting.

The dynamics within your family also play a significant role. Educating your family about ADHD fosters empathy and support, creating a nurturing home environment. Encourage siblings to be understanding and supportive, and involve them in the journey. It's also important to look after your well-being. Parenting a child with ADHD can be demanding, so self-care and seeking support when needed is crucial for maintaining your resilience and capacity to provide the best care for your child.

Remember, parenting a child with ADHD is a continual learning process. New challenges may arise, and strategies need to be adapted. Stay informed, be open to learning, and don't hesitate to ask for help when needed. With each step, you're not only helping your child manage their ADHD but also empowering them to discover their strengths and potential.

Finally, embrace this journey with positivity and hope. Children with ADHD possess unique talents and perspectives. They can navigate challenges and harness their strengths with your support, understanding, and advocacy. Your role as an advocate is not just about addressing difficulties but also about celebrating successes, big and small.

Your journey with ADHD is not one you walk alone. By integrating medical, educational, communal, and familial support, you create a robust network that surrounds your child with love, understanding, and opportunities for growth. It's this holistic approach that will enable your child with ADHD to thrive and achieve their fullest potential.

Conclusion

In this book, we have thoroughly examined a wide array of techniques and insights essential for parenting children with ADHD. We have covered everything from grasping the intricate aspects of ADHD, to valuing your child's individuality, and from enhancing communication skills to creating an environment at home that supports their needs.

Each chapter has been meticulously crafted to guide and strengthen you in your role as a parent. Alongside these strategies, we've discussed the significance of identifying and fostering your child's natural abilities, effectively handling ADHD in the presence of other conditions, and the pivotal influence of family relationships in bolstering your child's development.

Children with ADHD indeed possess remarkable potential. They are capable of leading rich and successful lives when provided with the appropriate support and understanding. This book aims to offer a beacon of hope and encouragement, emphasizing that ADHD is not a determinant of your child's future. Rather, it forms a part of their distinctive path, which, under your care and guidance, can lead to a life brimming with accomplishments and happiness.

Through the pages of this book, we aim to shift the focus from the challenges of ADHD to the opportunities it presents, helping parents to nurture these young minds into thriving individuals.

Embarking on the journey of parenting a child with ADHD is one marked by continual learning, steadfastness, and unconditional love. The strategies and insights detailed in this book are more than just advice; they are your companions along this path. It's essential to remember that each child is distinct, and their experience with ADHD is equally unique.

Embrace each obstacle as a chance to strengthen and deepen your bond with your child, transforming challenges into moments of joint triumph. The journey of parenting a child with ADHD is one of transformation and growth for both you and your child. Embrace it with an open heart and mind, and let this book be your guide and companion as you navigate this rewarding path.

Your Review Matter!

Congratulations on completing this journey into the world of ADHD parenting! You've unlocked a treasure trove of strategies and insights to achieve a positive mindset. But don't let the journey end with you. You have the power to light the way for others seeking the same transformation.

Your honest review can be the guiding star for those navigating the sea of books on Amazon. When you share your experience reading **ADHD Parenting Made Simple**, you're not just writing a review; you're extending a hand to someone who needs help parenting their ADHD child.

Think about it - your few simple words could be the push someone needs to help their child navigate this world with their challenging condition. Every act of sharing knowledge is a step toward helping a poor ADHD child. By leaving your review, you're joining us in a mission to tackle and defeat this increasing problem of ADHD.

So, please make a difference:

Scan the QR CODE below to leave your review on Amazon.

It's more than just a review; it's your legacy in the world of ADHD parenting.

Thank you for being an integral part of our journey and for helping others find their path to a happier, more positive life.

Sources

Archer, D. (2016). The ADHD Advantage: What You Thought Was a Diagnosis May Be Your Greatest Strength. Avery Publishing.

Baker, J. (2001). The Social Skills Picture Book: Teaching Communication, Play, and Emotion. Future Horizons.

Barkley, R. A. (2020). Taking Charge of ADHD: The Complete, Authoritative Guide for Parents. Guilford Press.

Barkley, R. A. (2015). Attention-Deficit Hyperactivity Disorder: A Handbook for Diagnosis and Treatment (4th ed.). Guilford Press.

Connor, D. F. (2015). Problems of overdiagnosis and overprescribing in ADHD. Psychiatric Times, 32(8).

Cooper-Kahn, J., & Dietzel, L. (2008). Late, Lost, and Unprepared: A Parents' Guide to Helping Children with Executive Functioning. Woodbine House.

Dawson, P., & Guare, R. (2009). Smart but Scattered: The Revolutionary 'Executive Skills' Approach to Helping Kids Reach Their Potential. Guilford Press.

Greene, R. W. (1998). The Explosive Child. HarperCollins Publishers.

Hallowell, E. M., & Ratey, J. J. (2011). Driven to Distraction: Recognizing and Coping with Attention Deficit Disorder. Anchor Publishing.

Ingersoll, B., & Dvortcsak, A. (2010). Teaching Social Communication to Children with Autism: A Practitioner's Guide to Parent Training. Guilford Press.

Jensen, P. S., & Cooper, J. R. (2002). Attention deficit hyperactivity disorder: State of the science-best practices (Vol. 7). Civic Research Institute.

Matthews, M., Nigg, J. T., & Fair, D. A. (2014). Attention

deficit hyperactivity disorder. Current Topics in Behavioral Neurosciences, pp. 16, 235–266.

Mayo Clinic Press. (n.d.). Busting ADHD myths: Helping parents better understand what ADHD can look like — and how it can be managed. Retrieved from https://mcpress. mayoclinic.org/blog/busting-adhd-myths-helping-parents-better-understand-what-adhd-can-look-like-and-how-it-can-be-managed/

Nadeau, K. G., & Quinn, P. O. (2002). Understanding women with AD/HD. Advantage Books.

Owens, E. B., Hinshaw, S. P., Lee, S. S., & Lahey, B. B. (2015). Journal of Clinical Child & Adolescent Psychology, 44(2), 199–211.

Pastor, P. N., Reuben, C. A., Duran, C. R., & Hawkins, L. D. (2015). NCHS Data Brief, (201), 1-8.

Rose-Krasnor, L., & Denham, S. (2009). Social-Emotional Competence in Early Childhood. In Handbook of Peer Interactions, Relationships, and Groups (pp. 162-179). Guilford Press.

Ratey, J. J., & Hallowell, E. M. (2008). Delivered from distraction: Getting the most out of life with attention deficit disorder. Ballantine Books.

Rief, S. F. (2016). The ADD/ADHD checklist: A practical reference for parents and teachers. Jossey-Bass.

Shapiro, L. E. (2010). The ADHD Workbook for Kids: Helping Children Gain Self-Confidence, Social Skills, and Self-Control. Instant Help: Edition 1

Visser, S. N., Danielson, M. L., Bitsko, R. H., Holbrook, J. R., Kogan, M. D., Ghandour, R. M., ... & Blumberg, S. J. (2015). Journal of the American Academy of Child & Adolescent Psychiatry, 54(1), 34-46.e2

MAKE SURE TO CHECK OUT
MY OTHER BOOK

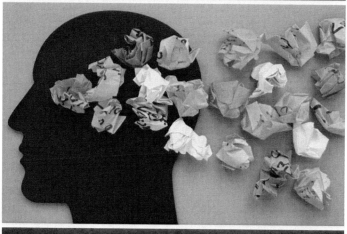

About the Author

Gregory Stide is a seasoned educator with over twenty years of experience teaching English to students from diverse backgrounds. His academic path began with a Bachelor's Degree in Computer Science, later enhanced by a Master's in English with a specialization in TESOL (Teaching English to Speakers of Other Languages). This unique combination of technological insight and linguistic skills has enabled him to create more accessible and engaging teaching methods, greatly benefiting students with varied learning styles.

Mr. Stide's career has been distinguished by his focus on adaptive teaching methods, particularly for students with learning differences such as ADHD. He strongly advocates for personalized educational approaches, believing them to be crucial for students with ADHD to achieve success. His experiences have proven that when teaching is tailored to individual needs, it can lead to significant improvements in learning outcomes.

In "ADHD Parenting Made Simple," Stide applies his extensive experience to offer parents practical insights and strategies for supporting children with ADHD. The book combines real-world teaching anecdotes with evidence-based techniques, emphasizing the importance of adaptability and understanding in educational methods. This guide aims to be a comprehensive resource for parents navigating the complex journey of ADHD parenting.

Gregory Stide is more than just an educator; he is an innovator in teaching strategies, especially for children with ADHD. His book "ADHD Parenting Made Simple" is a reflection of his dedication to education, showcasing his commitment to meeting the diverse needs of students. This work stands as a testament to his extensive teaching experience, offering invaluable guidance to parents and educators alike in the field of ADHD.

Manufactured by Amazon.ca
Acheson, AB